nelly grosjean

AROMATHERAPY

ESSENTIAL OILS FOR YOUR HEALTH

Also by nelly grosjean (all in French):

Aromathérapie, soigner grâce aux essences de plantes.
Chiron publishers.

Aromathérapie 2. Des huiles essentielles pour votre santé.
Vie Arôme publishers.

"Aromathérapie esthétique, des huiles essentielles beauté-santé."
Vie Arôme publishers.

"Aromathérapie des huiles essentielles dans votre assiette." L'alimentation gagneur.
Vie Arome publishers.

"Aromathérapie vétérinaire": in the course of being printed.

Illustrations, drawings and photographs by Marc Benedetti and Nelly Grosjean

SUMMARY OF CONTENTS

Introduction / History / Definitions

Chapter 1 THERAPY. Different uses of Essential Oils. Daily aromatic Files.

Chapter 2 THERAPY. Charts and classifications.

Chapter 3 Essential Oils for beauty.

Chapter 4 Essential Oils in the kitchen : cooking.

Architect of his own body
Man alone is fully responsible
For his own health.

HEALTH
IS AN
EQUILIBRIUM
between

what is absorbed

air
water
food
thought

what is eliminated

breathing out
urine
stools
relaxation

FOREWORD

Natural health advocates have been waiting a long time for a synthesis of this science,which is also a major art, deriving from orthodox naturopathy: aromatherapy.

nelly grosjean is one of the major contemporary specialists in aromatherapy*. Her reputation and expertise has crossed the Atlantic. This dictionary of aromatherapy is an essential tool for anyone wanting a serious but practical reference tool and guidelines on the application of this wonderful technique of natural health..

Today many para-naturopathic and eclectic methods attempt to invade the natural health field. but they lack a clear and synthetic approach. This could only come from an orthodox and highly respected naturopath who was trained in the best schools. nelly grosjean has produced an accurate and honest book which takes the art of aromatherapy out of the realm of improvisation and confusion.nelly grosjean's imposing work is a book to be contended with.

I hope that this dynamic, enthusiastic and competent woman will play an important role in the evolution of orthodox naturopathy which is the only global and fundamental medicine.

On behalf of my North American, European and international colleagues, I congratulate nelly grosjean on the publication of this work which marks an important date in the evolution of her profession and the health of mankind.

Dr. Jean-Marc BRUNET N.D., D.Sc., Ph.D.
Rector, Susan B Anthony University (U.S.A.)

*Nelly Grosjean, N.D., Doctor of Naturopathy, Susan B Anthony University, Missouri, U.S.A.

5

AROMATHERAPY

In England, aromatherapy is used by physiotherapists as a massage technique with the help of essential oils..(E.O.) An aromatherapist is therefore a physiotherapist.

In France , aromatherapy deals with the treatment of ailments through E.O.

The aromatherapist is a doctor or health practitioner who does not apply massages.

DEFINITIONS

AROMATHERAPY IS ETYMOLOGICALLY THE TREATMENT OF AILMENTS (THERAPY) WITH AROMAS (ESSENCES OR E.O. OF AROMATIC PLANTS).

AROMATHERAPY IS ONE OF THE TECHNIQUES OF HOLISTIC, ALTERNATIVE OR NATURAL MEDICINE.

AROMATHERAPY CAN BE AS MUCH PREVENTIVE AS CURATIVE.

AROMATHERAPY ABOVE ALL, "CURES", STRAIGHTENS AND RE-BALANCES THE WHOLE BODY.

"Germs are nothing,
the body is everything."
C. Bernard.

THE TEN GOLDEN RULES
FOR "LIVING WELL".

*Respect is the superior form
for the realisation of being.
It is reached only through knowing oneself.*

I have always been attached to these "golden rules for living well" and it seems normal to list them again at the start of this book. They never change and only practice allows positive consequences to act upon our physical, mental and spiritual well being.

Presented simply, clearly and precisely as a set of golden rules, here are the aromatherapic precepts and essential principles for good life hygiene.

They have to be applied daily to maintain your "health" capital, to avoid disease, to increase your own vital energy and your source of dynamism and "joie de vivre".

These golden rules can be applied to children, parents, adults, well or sick people and men and women. They are meant to improve the quality of life and bring healthy and often new habits into your home.

THE TEN GOLDEN RULES OF HEALTH AND BEAUTY

by nelly grosjean

1 - alimentation

2 - respiration

3 - physical exercise

4 - relaxation

5 - sleep

6 - importance of water

7 - sun

8 - sexual and affective balance

9 - aromatherapy

10 - positive thought

- An healthy and well-balanced alimentation
  Think raw. single meal, quietness
  Good elimination : drink to eliminate
  Supress the word "diet" of your vocabulary

- Breathe deeply during 3 minutes morning and evening
  and as often as possible all day long

- A few gymnastic exercises each day or practise a sport
  of your choice several times-a-week. Do it
  progressively with a "relaxation-recuperation"
  following time.

- 5 to 10 mn of relaxation will recharge your energy
  Sleep hours before midnight are double

- A cool shower every morning
  A warm shower or bath every evening

- Have "air" bathes and sun bathes as often as possible
  Favour your couple harmony each day

- Breathe an aromatised air with the aroma diffusor and
  have aromatic frictions every morning and evening

- Smile to yourself every single morning Have one
  positive action and one positive thought each day, at
  least

MEMENTO
HYGIENE FOR A HEALTHY LIFE

All species in life are in direct relation with the movement of the universe. through their structures, their forms and their tissues.

NUTRITION
1. EAT HEALTHY PRODUCTS,
whenever possible, additive and chemical free.
- Raw fresh vegetables in quantity, rather than cooked, vegetable juices, in quantity.
- Raw fresh fruit, always outside meals.
Without prior food, 10 am and 4 pm are the ideal times to eat raw fruit
Cooked fruit (stewed or even oven-cooked apples without sugar make excellent puddings)
- One protein per meal: egg, fish, poultry, meat, milk-based dish, or cereals.
- Good quality seasonings: cold, first pressed oils, sea salt, lemon or cider vinegar, natural yoghurts, cream cheeses.

2. TAKE THE TIME TO HAVE A MEAL, if possible in a calm environment.

3. REMEMBER TO CHEW and salivate.

4. WATCH FOR GOOD ELIMINATION.

5. DRINK AT LEAST 1 1/2 LITRES OF WATER PER DAY, outside meals; water or warm or cold infusion (Evian, Volvic).

DIET: Errors and food to avoid.

a) Number one enemy: sugar and its derivatives: sweets, chocolate, cakes, syrups and ice creams. Sugar from fruit taken daily is sufficient to satisfy our needs.

b) Bread, rice, pasta, white flour: wholly devitalised food. You could make wallpaper glue with their starch! Imagine the consequences for your organism.

c) Industrial preserves, delicatessen, cooked, prepared meals; heavy to digest, too often seasoned with a chemical sauce!

d) Wines, spirits, tea and coffee are stimulants turning into drugs. The habit should be broken!

e) Avoid too much meat: twice a day is too much!

f) Avoid too much cheese. It breeds rhumatism!

HISTORY OF AROMATHERAPY

The force which has created us and makes .
us live can also heal us.
(A Brazilian healer's saying)

In 1984 in different parts of the world researchers arrived at the following discoveries:
- DNA synthesis
- Discovery of life atom and death atom.
- Discovery of the cell sensitive to electromagnetic waves.
- Discovery of many synthetic drugs made from one of the scientifically isolated and active elements of a plant.
- Discovery "a posteriori" of the secondary reactions of the human body to synthetic drugs. Some of them found to be dangerous 30 years after their intensive use (DDT, Thalidomide).
- Discovery of the manifest activity of the many elements which make up a plant. The active principle, when isolated, does not show the same properties as the whole plant from which it is extracted.

Computer science opens up huge and brand new possibilities in medical investigation, chemistry, biology and pharmacology.Since the beginning of time plants have been widely used in the treatment of health. The World Health Organisation (WHO) has stated that many studies should be undertaken based on the knowledge of healers, herbalists and sorcerers all over the world so that scientific tests can be carried out to corroborate their empirical knowledge (1983,WHO statement)

Let's discover the history of plants and essential oils by travelling through time, civilisations and different world regions.

IN INDIA
The first medical document, Tsacharaka-Samhida, dates back to a 1,000 years BC.

The Artharweda, a major book which is still consulted, talks of plants breathing (respiration) energies. Medical treatments were collected there after the Aryan invasions.

IN CHINA

Tradition tells us that the God Emperor Shgen Nung 2838 to 2698 BC),
who ruled China, gave men botanical science.

Confucius (approx. 551 - 479 BC) the most famous of Chinese
philosophers, praises "the theory of vital energy and of breathing",
writes "the treatise of the bedroom", concerning hygiene and sexual
harmony, creates laws on hygiene, the salutary use of baths, showers,
massages and tells us that "coitus" means "battle of flowers".

Tsao-Tchouan (approx 540 BC) and the Han Dynasty relate to
medicine "beyond the Century of Iron, to the Saints and Sages of the
Golden Age".

During the Mandarin era "a great physician does not treat what is
already sick, he treats that which is not yet". (Old Chinese saying)

IN EGYPT

Marjoram is attributed to Osiris, armoise to Isis, marrube to Horus,
and camomile to the Sun.

The medicinal principles of pharaonic Egypt are gathered in the "Ebers"
papyri found in Thebes in 1873. At any given time , the miracle cure is
being searched for: Polydamno finds the "magical sap, pain and anger
soothing, which makes forget all ailments". Papyri dating back to 2800
BC testify to that:

"origano, cinnamon, juniper and mint were part of ointments and
creams prepared from the squeezing out of the essence of herbs or their
maceration in fat oil".

"In temples, precious ointments and fragrant essences".
Fragrant essences were used to embalm high ranking Egyptians.

Preparation of essences, oils and flowers, 2800 BC the era of the first
squeezed out plants in Egypt.

IN GREECE

Theophraste wrote "the treatise of odours" Is this a departure or a continuity of Aromatherapy through the ages?

Chiron, sage and centaurus, cures Phoenix' cecity with medicinal plants one of which is centaurea. At the time, Asklepios, the Greek god of medicine heals with "words, simples and a blade", so says Pindarus. Hence Asclepiades meaning physician-priests. According to " the history of Medicine" the methods are primitive, limited only to a few traditional phytotherapeutic, or elementary physiological means and some surgery.

Was Heraclius the first hygienist?

Hercules advocated warm hydrotherapy and simples, and Melampsus King of Pylos and a physician, already practised metallotherapy by curing Iphides of his impotence with iron oxide.

Esculapus, a physician and the son of Apollo, himself the God of Medicine, could raise the dead. Maybe his status as the son of God had given him Jesus Christ's powers.

Panaceus was a renowned healer from whom derived the word panacea, a universal remedy. Panaceus also represented a Greek goddess, the daughter of Esculapus and grand-daughter of Apollo.

Hippocrates (Vth century BC) is the father of medicine as we all know it. His famous oath is still taken by doctors at the start of their careers.

Aristotle and Theophraste were his students. Dioscorides (1st century BC) exerted the greatest influence upon botanists of the Renaissance. Plinius and Galienus succeeded Dioscorides and increased the sum of his work.

In Greece, "Treatise of Odours" by Theophraste.

IN PERSIA

Avicenne (980 AC) in his own "Canon of Medicine" relates that "whilst studying medical plants, he discovers the method to prepare volatile essences of flowers and plants through distillation". The "Canon of medicine" by Avicenne became, at the time, the reference work for Muslims and Westerners.

In Persia, Avicenne became the inventor of distillation.

IN ROME

Aromatic oils were part of youth elixirs and Hercules' sacred plant was the poplar;

IN THE MIDDLE AGES

Physicians were still priests. Pope Innocent 111 decreed a papal law by which no ecclesiast was allowed to practise medicine for money nor shed any blood at all. Physician monks thus began cultivating herbal gardens, became apothecaries (they left their Orders) of healers who sold their potions from towns to villages. Physician-priests who remained within the Church's fold bestowed their medical duties on to barbers, as the physician diagnosed without touching the patient, but through his urine and his horoscope. he then sent his instructions to the apothecary. the treatment of the sick took into account the writings of Hippocrates which contained the four constitutions: sanguine, phlegmatic, bilious, melancholic. the four moods: blood, Air - phlegm, Water - bile, Fire - atrabilious, Earth. In China it was based on Yin and Yang and the theory of the five elements.

The XVIth century sees the doctrine of similars (law of similtude), the search for a treatment in the cause of illness: one of the bases of Homeopathy.

The majority of drugs are vegetable based and alchemistry allows for great progress in chemistry and metallurgy. The search for the eternal life elixir has always given scholars an occasion to surpass themselves.

The external and internal use of aromatic herbal oils figure in some texts from the XVIth century and before. and is identical to what we know today of Aromatherapy.

Essential Oils are then considered as the pure spirit of a plant and therefore act through thought and emotions, and on the external body. dew from herbs, special breathing and exercising methods, were used and music was considered particularly beneficial, Alto - Tenor - Bass - Soprano, placed in parallel with the four moods.

Preventative medicine was also predominant, especially where diets were concerned following Hippocrates' good old principle: " Let food be your medicine".

Aromatic essential Oils
for external or internal use, are, in the Middle Ages
"the pure spirit of a plant."

Little by little, medicine and botany progress as the power of the Church on physicians decreases.

THEN CAME THE XXth CENTURY
The awakening of modern medicine, the famous work of P. and M. Curie, C. Bernard and Pasteur with his astonishing sentence:
"Germs are nothing, the body is all", demonstrate the new road to follow: the study and knowledge of the body present as much interest, if not more, than the study of germs .....

But one has to go very far back in time to discover the real premisses for today's naturopathic medicine, the treatment for a whole person. In fact we have to go back to the Sumerian.

50 CENTURIES AGO
Surgeons, herbalists, naturopaths and priests were learned physicians who treated "the spirit to heal the body", and discovered that "darkness (the word "illness" did not exist) was a "curative crisis" in preparation for the birth of the Spirit. (Document found on the site of the ruined Sumerian city of Nippur)

Sumerian sacred medicine, according to Maguerite Enderlin, an eminent French sumerologist, recounts astonishing elements which tend to prove that all the practitioners and naturopaths in "soft" medicine had famous precursors: scholars who worked in astrology, phytotherapy, anatomy, pharmacopea, diagnoses and prognoses, the practice of hepatoscopy, secret sciences which gave them the ability to interpret dreams, colours, oil stains on water.

The Sumerian physician-priest was a miracle worker who knew how to escort his patient down and back from hell.
The secret and initiatory teaching passed on to each Sumerian physician has not yet been deciphered from tablets and perhaps it will remain thus forever unbroken.

Following a spiritual preparation based on meditation and prayers, the Sumerian physician started with a clinical examination of the patient, his stature, gait, aggressivity, mental disorders, temperature, eye quality, retina, urine, elasticity of muscles, small, then observation and deduction from the state of organs and analysis of internal pains, lastly, examination of head and bones.

The Sumerian physician knew the importance of aggravating or improving rhythms and administered his medication at set , times - at dawn, twilight or at night, according to each case.

Other stone tablets mention the critical periods of any given disease and its cyclic or successive phases and predict the number of days between a fatal issue or full recovery. On some tablets dating back over 4000 years, diagnoses and medical prescriptions can also be found.

Frictions and inhalations with essences
were practised over 4000 years ago!

Aromatherapy, oligosols and lithotherapy (grounded stones) were used currently in Sumer in the remotest Antiquity, in treatments where all techniques co-habited and where physicians were "specialists in all matters", practising medicine for the whole person, physical, spiritual and holistic ....

At this level, the new orthodox naturapath doctors, be they energeticians, acupuncturists, psychomatricians or hypnotizers, met up with Sumerian sacred medicine. Only a few years ago we ignored that frictions with essential oils were currently used in those days to maintain good health, re-establish the proper circulation of the "breath of life" = vital energy, to favour "re-vitalisation" = healing. The role of the Sumerian physician was to allow his patient to recover "the light of glory" and "the heart's secret" = good health! The evolution of man between his stages of "light" = good health and "darkness" = disease, allowed him to get closer to immortality This state of equilibrium is close to Hindu and Tibetan writings on the eternal evolution of Being, through moral and physical trials.

The Sumerian physician, the Tibetan lama and Muslim priests were bestowed with this high and glorious task: to help man in his spiritual progress, thanks to the maintenance of his physical state and of his psyche.
Let's hope the doctors do not forget the full and whole dimension of their task; only then shall we benefit from whole medicine, a medicine for Man in his full spiritual and physical entity, and not a medicine of symptoms, which cuts man up in slices, and where each specialist heals only the parts he has elected to treat .....

A medicine unified over the whole body, a medicine of physical, psychic, and spiritual bodies. Tomorrow's medicine towards which we are progressing in great strides for everyone's good.

A human medicine!
Orthodox Naturopathy!
Holistic medicine!

And finally the most ancient relationship between man and plants : over 60,000 years ago, primitive man buried his dead covered with flowers ! (excavation of the Shanidar caves).

personal notes

ESSENTIAL OIL (E.O)
Definition

Essential Oil (E.O.) is the noble (or first) yield from the distillation of an aromatic plant. The aromatic plant contains sufficient quantities of aromatic and odoriferous principles in order to be distilled.

Not all plants yield essential oils. However, all plants can be distilled so that only the floral water, hydrosol or hydrolat, can be produced.

Hydrosol or hydrolat is the complementary yield to EO. It is obtained by distilling a plant. It contains a minute proportion of suspended aromatic principles and in sufficient quantity to generate therapeutic actions.

Hydrosol-therapy is slightly similar to aromatherapy's homeopathy. Often used in drinks and healthcare products, it adapts itself perfectly to infants, sensitive, even fragile, persons and /or aggravated, objective or subjective, reactions. For example:
"I do not want to absorb EO. It burns. It's too strong"."When I absorb them I belch. I feel as if my stomach is burning" ..... etc

Aromatherapy and hydrosoltherapy act primarily on a daily diet. How?

- in seasonings (salads, sauces, cereals)
- in drinks (hot or cold)
- in a diet of healthy drinking : the "health" drinks
- in treatment: "cocktails", "toddies" ....

HYDROSOL: HOMEOPATHY OR ALCHEMY OF AN AROMA

Definition

Hydrosol is "our" designation for hydrolat or floral water from a distillation with spring water and of which only the first 20 litres are collected. During distillation, heated water passes steam through plants carrying aromatic principles with it before it is cooled. The essential oil is separated from the floral water through a density differential in the distiller.

Hydrosol from all existing plants can be obtained, even from the non-aromatic ones (oak, beech, fenugreek, holly, boxwood, plantain, fern), but only "aromatic" plants will yield essential oil.

The aromatic principles suspended in water, together with water produce an hydrolat. As soon as these aromatic principles are in quantities sufficient to be separated from water, they create the essential oil, or essence, which floats on the surface of the distillation water. Aromatic molecules merge according to their own quantity to create aromatic essential oil.

The plant's aromatic principle comes from small "aroma bags" in aromatic plants which are "exploded" in the distilling process. Steam precipitates them in the distillation water from which they will be separated by the essence distiller.

In the case of citrus fruit, these "aroma bags" can also be opened mechanically (i.e. the zest from: lemon, orange, bergamot, mandarin and grapefruit).

SYNERGY

Synergy is the association of several factors whose coordinated action creates a single effect.

The therapeutic potential of natural products is sublimated by synergy.

Synergy is the source of additional and mysterious properties which cannot be wholly explained by mathematical addition.

The synergy of essential oils therefore creates a "new product" with different properties and for which therapeutic possibilities happened to be more important, more selective and more efficient or simply different ....

1 + 1 + 3 and more and more ....

N.B. For prescriptions on the following pages, i.e. internal absorption :
Essential Oil (1 to 3 drops) can be taken on a honey spoonful or in a glass of hot, not, boiling water.

The ideal is to place a drop of essential Oil on the back of your hand and to lick it up. This is an easy and practical method for a thorough treatment in the office or when travelling.

THE PLATEAU EFFECT*

One of the things upon which I shall insist the most is the importance of using small doses, short cures and the indispensable change of E.O.

During an aromatherapeutic treatment course, following the ensuing modifications to the body. Thanks to E.O., these occur rapidly. This is confirmed by the plateau effect: the physiological response to any given medication. Prescribed doses will bring proportional results to a given threshold, defined and variable according to the E.O. used. If the prescribed dose increases in quantity or is cumulative, the results, until then proportional, will be inverted: the response, that is the expected therapeutic effect, thus becomes negative, even opposite.

Throughout this book, I advise against the "blind" use of E.O. and against the noxious effects of heavy doses. It would therefore be wise to respect the doses recommended for given pathological cases or advised for preventive indications.

Summary: Low doses
            + short treatments
            + change and adjustments of E.O.
            as treatment proceeds
            _____
            = Expected therapeutic result.

* Named after the person who discovered the "Plateau" effect.
E.O.= Essential oil

They aim at favouring, in the home, the practical and intelligent use of essential oils for parents concerned with the proper application of aromatherapy and a new and healthy way of life:

To maintain and increase
everyone's "health" capital.

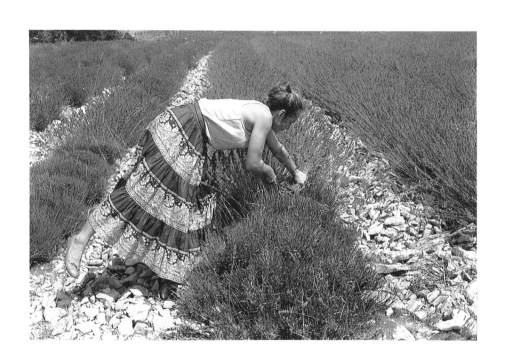

nelly grosjean collecting lavender with a pruning knife, at an altitude of 1,100 metres . This biological crop is cultivated by Vie' Arôme. France.

CHAPTER I

THERAPY

- diffusion

- frictions

- internal uses

- inhalations

- baths

- other uses.

Anyone who takes care of his
breathing brings Order within
his Self
Poa P'outseu.

DIFFUSION IN THE ATMOSPHERE

Aromatic essential oils diffused in the atmosphere thanks to a diffuser, allow the "absorption through the lungs" of volatile micro-particles - the active principles - of essential oils.

The diffusion of E.O. in the atmosphere is the first and best way to benefit from essential oils, without any inconvenience.

ACTION OF ESSENTIAL OILS IN THE ATMOSPHERE

a) Eliminate any unpleasant smell
Tobacco - smoke - crowd - sanitary - cooking......

b) Revitalize - Rejuvenate - Re-energetize the air you breathe.

c) Offer negative ions.
So often absent from cities and dwellings, this influx of negative ions is less important through the diffusion of essential oils in the atmosphere than through the negative ions generator. It is however sufficiently and harmoniously completed by the specific properties of essential oils.

d) Offer the specific properties of essential oils
through smelling, breathing the following essential oils :

Respiratory

Pine, Eucalyptus, Cajeput, Niaouli, Thyme, Hyssop, Lavender

Revitalising

Coriander, Savory, Nutmeg, Rosemary, Clove, Origano, Rose, Geranium.

Relaxing
Lavender, Marjoram, Camomile, Orange, Petit-Grain, Neroli, Bergamot.

Exotic Revitalising
Cinnamon, Sandal Wood, Ylang-Ylang.

Soft and Pleasant
Vervain, Rose geranium, Rosewood, Camomile.

THE AROMA DIFFUSER

This is an electrical tool which allows the dispersion of micro-particles of essential oils in the atmosphere through vibrations. Thanks to this method essential oils are not heated and therefore maintain all their properties.

Essential oils placed in the specially designed glassware nebulise in the room where the diffuser is placed.

It functions:
- with a reduced volume : all day or all night.
- with a maximum volume : 1 hr. in the morning and 1 hr. in the evening before going to bed.

Various models are adapted to the size of rooms.

Advantages of the electrical aroma diffuser
- Essential oils are not heated.
- In record time - approx. 15 mins - the air of a room is saturated with essential oils.
- The practical side of the aroma diffuser: it can use different compositions for day or night, for colder days, or simply for the comfort of your home.

Functioning duration of the aroma diffuser
- In the house : You switch on for 1 hour in the morning and 1 hour at night at maximum volume or else all day or all night at minimum volume.
- In a conference room : Switch on to maximum throughout the conference.

- In an office, shop, hotel lobby, doctor's room, reception rooms : The equipment can function non-stop.

- To sleep better : Switch on for 1 hour in the room before going to bed.

- During winter : Switch on, non-stop, in the living rooms.

INCENSE BURNERS : Berger Lamps
Scent the atmosphere but do not have an important therapeutic action. However, the diffusion of essential oils through this means purifies the atmosphere whilst making it pleasant.

A FEW DROPS OF ESSENTIAL OILS ON LAMPS OR SAUCERS

On a radiator, they cleanse and scent the atmosphere, in a simple, practical and cheap way, especially in winter with respiratory essential oils - or in summer on lamps with essential oils against mosquitoes.

POT POURRI DIFFUSER

In a pretty bowl filled with dried flowers add a few drops of your essential oils (approx.100 drops = 1 small spoon, monthly)

In summary: The breathing of essential oils-charged air would be sufficient to avoid many epidemics, chills, would be conducive to relaxation and energy and would help to introduce cellular harmony into your body: Factor of good health - Joie de vivre, happiness!
"Bonheur"

IN DIFFUSION, THE MOST EXOTIC APPRECIATED ESSENTIAL OIL :

The essential oil of "bonheur"; Vervain is always much loved by all in any circumstances.

The list of essential oils which are pleasant when diffused is to be found in the table "Use of the main essential oils".

You will find Respiratory, Relaxing, Tonic, Aphrodisiacal, Harmonious, Exotic compositions in the various files on essential oils.

There are many recipes for excellent compositions in the following chapters:
Cajeput; Camomile, Cedar, Coriander, Eucalyptus, Rose, Geranium, Hyssop, Lavender, Marjoram, Mint, Orange, Origano, Rosemary, Sage, Thyme, Vervain.

We can stop eating for thirty days,
We can stop drinking for three days,
But we cannot stop breathing for over three minutes!
Hence the importance of breathing and , furthermore of a
good, revitalised, re-energitised air thanks to essential oils.

FRICTIONS WITH AROMATIC OILS *

When the Egyptians started using essential oils, in addition to embalments, it was through frictions. they appreciated those for their fragrance as much as for their properties.

This mixture is really the origin of perfume ! Perfumes were a mixture of essential oils prepared according to the wishes and tastes of each and everyone and for specific frictions.

WHY USE ESSENTIAL OIL IN FRICTIONS

We know that after applying essential oils on the skin, they penetrate the blood and lymph within four hours.

Furthermore, the exceptional and selective property of essential oils offers the following advantage :

essential oils in frictions on any part of the body will inevitably be attracted by the weak organ or the perturbed function.

General precaution: avoid mucous membrane and genital parts.

We shall first discuss the "health frictions" which anyone should apply to increase his vital potential and which help the body to awake in the morning and relax and sleep well at night.

- Tonic frictions
- Relaxing frictions
- Digestive frictions
- Respiratory frictions
- Circulatory frictions
- "anti-pain" frictions
- Aphrodisiac frictions

* See "Frictions" with essential oils in chapter 3

Then the following specific frictions:

- Skin frictions
- Foot frictions(with foot massage)
- Hair frictions

General dosage

Body frictions	30 drops
Stomach and abdomen frictions	10 to 20 drops.
Pains frictions	5 to 10 drops.
Legs frictions	10 to 20 drops.
Feet frictions	10 drops.
Hair frictions	50 to 100 drops.
Face frictions	5 to 7 drops.
Chest and back frictions	20 to 30 drops.

For children with very delicate skin:
Frictions are always mixed with an identical volume of wheatgerm, sweet almond or olive oil.

SPECIAL PRECAUTIONS

**NEVER APPLY FRICTIONS ON INFANTS
(6 months or younger)..**

In aromatherapy, we prefer small, regular doses...
and cure courses of 3 to 6 weeks...

Only a few essential oils can be used as such or in composition, without being diluted.

The other essential oils must be mixed with at least one of the oils listed below in small quantity, or mixed with wheat germ, sweet almond or olive oil, in a neutral body milk or lastly in essential oil of lavender.

Natural & non-diluted	Mixed or diluted...
Rosewood	Green Anise
Cajeput	Basilic
Camomile	Bergamot
Caraway	Cinnamon
Cedar	Coriander
Lemon	Tarragon
Cypress	Ginger
Eucalyptus	Clove
Juniper	Lemongrass
Rose Geranium	Mint
Lavender	Nutmeg
Marjoram	Neroli
Niaouli	Origano
Orange	Rose
Petit Grain	Savory
Pine	Sassafras
Rosemary	Sage
Sandalwood	Turpentine
Ylang-Ylang	Thuya
	Thyme
	Vervain

Special precautions : with Mint, Thyme, Origano, Clove, Ginger which will enter - maximum 1/10 - in compositions.

Finally the mixing of essential oils will have to be followed carefully as indicated further.

A few methods exist but in any case it is advisable to :

- never mix more than three essential oils together (unless you have intimate knowledge of their respective synergies) (see: Synergies, definition, or follow the advice of your aromatherapist).

- refer strictly to the specific indications given in this book.

Example : for a respiratory problem.
It's better to a have a good eucalyptus friction alone than an erroneous mixture of all essential oils labelled "respiratory".

The efficiency of any mixture is often inferior to the use of one single essential oil.

WHEN TO APPLY FRICTIONS

Morning, between 6 am and midday	Morning tonics
Evening, between 6 pm and midnight	Evening relaxation
5 pm and before going to bed	Aphrodisiacs
10 am, 4 pm and before going to bed	Circulatory
After your three meals	Digestive
Morning and evening	Respiratory
Morning, 5 pm and before going to bed	Circulatory
Morning and evening	Feet

HOW TO APPLY FRICTIONS

First method: take a few drops of the chosen composition on your hand.
Rub the two hands and spread on treated parts the rotating of massage-friction clockwise.

Second method: Put the drops on the parts to be treated
and rub as above.

WHERE TO APPLY FRICTIONS

On the whole body :

Chest, neck, spine, arms, legs, soles of feet and solar plexus.	Tonic Relaxing Aphrodisiacs
Chest, back and solar plexus	Respiratory
Stomach, abdomen and solar plexus	Digestive
Any painful part and solar plexus	Anti-pain
Feet, legs and solar plexus	Circulatory
Feet only	Foot
Scalp	Hair
Face only	Face

The last three are more relevant to a "cosmetic" than an
"aromatherapeutic" application.
For shingles, eczema, scabies and most dermatoses,
frictions are more efficient when - with the same specific
composition - a friction on the solar plexus is added.

MAIN PRINCIPLES
General Dosage
INTERNAL USES

- 1 to 3 drops of essential oils or mixture, 2 to 5 times per day, are the average dosage - except special prescription.

- Course treatments of up to 3 weeks maximum of the same essential oil or mixture.

Directions for use:
In the past it was recommended that essential oils be taken on sugar. This was a very bad habit since sugar, even brown, is a "poison" for the nervous cell.

We recommend taking essential oils in a sugar substitute - honey, a good vehicle for the absorption and assimilation of essential oils.

The second best way to absorb essential oils is to take them in a large glass of warm water.They do not mix or dilute in water. However from the three prescribed drops, only half or one drop will remain in the glass and not be absorbed. The rest will be swallowed.

How to take essential oils: 7 good methods:

1) Place on the back of the hand, 1 to 3 drops of essential oil and lap, then drink a large glass of warm water, an infusion or eat a large spoonful of honey or yoghurt to "get rid of the taste".

2) Take 1 to 3 drops on a spoonful of good quality honey not heated.

3) Take 1 to 3 drops in a large glass of warm water or hot water: it should not be boiling, as the volatile and subtle aromatic principles of the essential oils deteriorate in the heat.

4) Drinks with essential oils. You will find the relevant recipes under the various headings for the following essential oils :

Anti-tobacco	Sassafras
Anti-flu	Origano, Thyme, Eucalyptus
Pleasant drinks	Lemon, Cedar
Drinks for indigestion	Origano
Memory cocktail	Ginger, Savory
Asthma cocktail	Thyme
Aphrodisiac drinks	Ginger, Savory

5) Pearls or capsules can also be prescribed by your aromatherapist. Capsules keep essential oils odourless and tasteless.

Intestinal capsules offer both inconvenience and advantages which your aromatherapist will weigh.

However, there is another handicap: the gustative wall no longer exists and they could, without apparent inconvenience, be taken in great quantities.

For example: nothing prevents you from taking ten capsules of Thyme at once - except your good sense - but it is really impossible to swallow 10 drops of essential oil of thyme, only one being already hard to ingest.

6) Essential oils in alcoholic solution can be prepared on prescription by your pharmacist.

7) Numerous essential oils can be used in cookery:

Thyme, Rosemary, Savory, Juniper, Caraway, Cumin, Nutmeg, Anise, Fennel, Coriander, Sage, Ginger: in, savoury dishes.

Lemon, Orange, Grapefruit, Mandarin, Cinnamon, Ginger, Rose Geranium : in sweet dishes.

Refer to a few good recipes at the end of this book : Chapter 4 : Essential oils in the kitchen.

If one remembers that getting close to a de-mineralised person will "relieve" you of your mineral salts in his/her favour. Therefore it should be sufficient to touch essential oils for them to be efficient.

Without going to the extreme of this empirical and esoteric, but not inaccurate theory, let's remember that the ingestion, the presence of essential oils, is preferable in small doses several times per day to a daily dose taken once. The results depend on the importance and regularity of treatments.

You will find in the glossary of this book precise instructions on essential oils and how to use them, according to illnesses. You will find tables and dosage, frequency and length of treatments in the corresponding files.

Nothing is lost
Nothing is created
All is transformation
Lavoisier
Alexis Carrel

ABSORPTION

1) Place I drop of E.O. on the back of the hand and lap: the simplest and most practical method.

2) For children : hydrosols (soft aromatherapy) or water from the distillation which contains suspended aromatic principles - to be preferred to essential oils, except on advice from the aromatherapist.

3) For infants : NEVER USE ANY ESSENTIAL OIL in internal treatment.
In friction, use hydrosols of lavender, pine, eucalyptus....

Never any essential oil frictions on infants

In prescriptions, they will always be diluted and mixed with wheat germ oil.
- lavender remains the infants' E.O., always diluted.
- for infants it is recommended to seek the advice of your holistic physician.

INHALATIONS - PREPARATION AND USE

Inhalation is one of the best practical means to benefit from essential oils associated to warm, relieving, steam.The inhalator allows for the breathing of warm vapours loaded with essential oils.

Inhalations are used mostly for respiratory and pulmonary infections, some migraines, headaches, mainly of a nervous or digestive origin.

Warmth relaxes.

The warm steam when breathed calms coughs, clears pulmonary tracks, soothes bronchial coughs, calms neuralgia. Essential oils offer their own specific properties.

Inhalations made with essential oils:

- **Soothing**   Lavender, Marjoram, Orange, Camomile.

- **Respiratory**   Pine, Eucalyptus, Niaouli, Cajeput, Lavender, Thyme, Rosemary, Hyssop, Origano.

Use

A few drops (3 to 10) of the chosen essential oils are placed in an inhalator, a large bowl, or even a saucepan of hot water.

Put your head above the inhalator or container, whilst covering your head with a large bath towel, so that the warm vapours are not dispersed but "inhalated".

Duration

Inhalations last 3 to 7 minutes, according to what is bearable, and can be renewed without trouble, 2, 3 or 4 times daily.

Flu, colds, chest infections, irritating coughs, bronchitis, asthma, tuberculosis and all respiratory infections, facial neuralgia, migraine and some cephalea. Inhalations will bring relief to all these.

Recipes
See Eucalyptus, Hyssop, Lavender, Rosemary and Thyme for dosage and specific instructions.

AROMATIC BATH WITH ESSENTIAL OILS

Cleopatra used to bathe in jenny's milk. Over the past centuries famous women took scented baths. Early in this century Abbot Kneipp treated mainly with all forms of hydrotherapy : warm or cold baths, ablutions, showers of all kinds. L. Kuhne cured many diseases by strengthening the body with hip baths frictions, feet, hands, trunk, baths ... Hence through the centuries:

The importance of water and its medicinal properties.

A healer after a seance, without having even touched his patient, washes his hands to rid himself of "negative or dirty vibrations" which he might have accumulated ...

Water washes the body and the spirit.

What's more relaxing than a bath or a shower after a day's work ? Not only water cleanses but it takes away the major part of "negative and invisible particles" which takes it back to the earth.....

We know about the great conductive, electrical power of water. Some masseurs work whilst keeping one of their hands connected to a copper wire - a power transmitter - or to a water mains. various esoteric writings note the importance of the ability water has to discharge negative "waves", electro-magnetic vibrations subjected to the same as electricity.

Have you ever realized that our thoughts are translated in space through *"vibrations"* or *"waves"* such as to be one day intercepted, in the same manner as radio or television waves are today?

Furthermore, water is a generator of *negative ions* vital to the equilibrium of the air, our first "food" for survival. Cities are overloaded with positive ions and only waterfalls, the sea, oceans, turbulent baths, *all live waters, fabricate negative ions....*

Many examples show the importance of water: Roman baths, hammams, Finnish saunas associated with cold baths, in an air charged with negative ions amongst the pine forests, Turkish baths, spa centres and today the craze for balneotherapy, thalassotherapy and the new Californian spa, the jacuzzi and bubble baths...

Any "naturapathic treatment" or "body shaping treatment" is based on a good food balance, an energetic equilibrium, and the elimination of toxins and deficiencies.

Baths with plants or even better aromatic baths, figure as the "Mighty Lords" at the heart of these treatments.

> *Saving water which washes the body*
> *and the spirit of all impurities.*

Let's add to these wonderful properties of water, the power of essential oils and then we have harmonising baths, physically and mentally, balancing baths for our perturbed energies, relaxing baths, tonic ones, energising ones.... baths for life!

OTHER USES

- Vaginal injections and enema
- Hair care
- Veterinary usage

REFLEXOTHERAPY

Essential oils have been used on acupuncture spots; aural acupuncture and digital acupuncture for some years. Research in these areas is still being carried out.
Firstly, specific essential oils on a strategic spot, increase the positive effects of relaxotherapy.
Essential oils "produce" a new energy.
Reflexotherapy "balance" these energies.
Aromatherapy and reflexotherapy both belong to:
Soft medicine, medicines of energies, tomorrow's medicines.

VETERINARY AROMATHERAPY

Our good friends cats , dogs, horses, ducks, geese .... can also benefit from the effects of aromatic essential oils. Many veterinary surgeons are nowadays practising aromatherapy. For cats and dogs an aroma diffuser with respiratory E.O. resorb respiratory problems. Diffusers can also be installed in stables, duck or geese ponds .....

For cats and dogs, frictions with E.O. will give good results. Did you know that osteopathy is also practised on animals? To deodorise an appartment where cats live: aroma diffuser with exotic vervain, mint tonic or frestonic. Immediate result.

With dogs, for a full hair, one tablespoon of yeast with all their meals, a course of chloride of magnesium 3 to 4 times per year (20 gr per litre of water, 1/2 glass twice a day) and frictions with E.O..

personal notes

personal notes

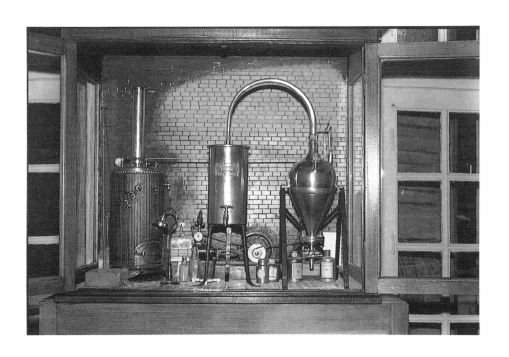

Miniature, distillation factory at the beginning of nineteenth century.

DAILY AROMATIC FILES

Presentation of aromatic files and how to use them

The aromatic files are shortened summaries.

You can take them around your home, in the kitchen or in the bathroom. They can be detached from the book and plasticized.

It is recommended that you follow the more developed and precise information which you will find throughout this book.

ABREVIATIONS

tble. sp.	table spoon	E.U.	External use
sm. sp.	Small spoonful	/week	Per week
1 x D.	Once a day	bef.	Before
Dur.	During	in	In
drp.	Drop	W.G.O.	Wheat germ oil
E.O.	Essential Oil	all	All
trt.	Treatment	O.of	Oil of
I.U.	Internal use	fw.	Few

CARAWAY
"E.O.. - FLATULENCE TYPE"

- **Intestinal oxygeniser, the best of all digestives.**
Flatulence, distending, and all dyspepsiae

DOSAGE
I.U. : 1 to 2 drops 3 x/day: AFTER MEALS on hand in water or honey.
E.U. : 5 to 10 drops as friction on stomach and abdomen. after meals.

Course: 3 x/day for 3 weeks   **PREVENTION:** 1 treatment 2 to 4 X/YEAR.

SYNERGIES - RECIPES
- I.U. + E.U.
1 drop caraway + 1 nutmeg 3 x/day after meals

- DIGESTIVE COMPOSITION
45 ml caraway + 30 nutmeg + 20 coriander + 5 cumin: a few drops as friction after meals or DIG friction.

- CULINARY AROMATHERAPY
caraway, cumin, coriander, nutmeg, juniper, thyme, tarragon, rosemary
1 to 2 drops in cooked dishes to enhance flavour (sauerkraut, stews, couscous)
E.O. IN DISHES HELP WITH DIGESTING HEAVY MEALS

- DIGESTIVE LIQUOR.
20 drops of caraway + 5 cumin + 5 geranium + 10 coriander + 2 nutmeg + 1 lavender in 1/2 litre alcohol(80°C) + 11/2 litres sugar syrup in mix still warm. (prepare syrup with 370 gms sugar for 1/2 litre distilled water, heat till transparent).
KEEP 15 TO 30 DAYS BEFORE DRINKING.

E.O. of Caraway is the "miracle" cure for flatulence.

CINNAMON
"E.O. - TYPE FOR DIARRHEA"

- **Strong antiseptic, stimulating, aphrodiasiac, antispasmodic.**
- Diarrhea, colitis, impotence and frigidity.

DOSAGE
I.U. : 1 drop 3 x/day on hand in water or honey
E.U. : frictions and baths
      always diluted in EO lavender of WGO.
Course: 3 to 4 x/day during crisis **PREVENTION:** 1 x/day for 3 weeks.

SYNERGIES - RECIPES

- APHRODISIAC FRICTION
  5 ml cinnamon + 10 coriander + 15 rosemary + 5 clove
  + 5 ginger + 15 marjoram or APH friction.
  twice a day on solar plexus, nape and spine.

- APHRODISIAC OIL
  7 ml cinnamon + 15 rosewood + 2 sandalwood or ylang-ylang in 100 ml WGO

- DIFFUSION IN ATMOSPHERE TO "EXOTISE" AIR
  10 ml cinnamon + 30 cedar + 60 lavender.

- PERFUME
  100 ml alcohol (70° C) + 10 cinnamon + 1 clary sage

- ANTI-FLU TODDY
  1 drop cinnamon + 1 origano + 1 thyme + 1 clove + 1 geranium
  + 1 ginger (optional) in sp/honey + very hot water + 1 lemon
  juice. Taste. You can drink 2/3 x/day without problem.

- APHRODISIAC COCKTAIL AND WONDERFUL INTELLECTUAL STIMULANT
  1 drop cinnamon (Ceylan) + 1 savory + 1 clove + 1 rosemary + 1
  geranium in a large glass of warm water, serve with ice cubes as a
  long drink. A dash of mint cordial can complete this cocktail or 1
  sm sp of hydrosol of mint.

NOTE : 1 drop of cinnamon every two hours, stops diarrhea.

*NEVER USE EO CINNAMON UNDILUTED IN BATH OR FRICTION
it would turn you into a fire! Cinnamon burns the skin.*

CAMOMILE
"E.O. - SINUSIS TYPE   ·

- Antispasmodic.
- Sinusitis, migraine, vertigo, dysmenorrhea, irritability, allergies.

DOSAGE
I.U.   : 1 drop 3 x/day in water or honey
E.U.   : Frictions 10 to 15 drops, on temples, forehead, nape, solar plexus and spine, 2 x/day.

Course: during biological disorder, a few days treatment I.U. + E.U.

PREVENTION: diffusion in atmosphere.

SYNERGIES - RECIPES

- SINUSITIS
  Camomile + lavender . Equal parts. 3 applications/day

- MIGRAINE, CEPHALEA, VERTIGO
  5 drops camomile + 5 marjoram + 5 mint, 2 massages/day on temples or HAR friction.

- SOOTHING BATH
  5 drops camomile + 5 lavender in 2 tble sp powdered milk or green seaweeds..

- DIFFUSION IN ATMOSPHERE
  . For allergies
  . To favour "harmony and creativity"
  camomile + rosewood + cedar. Equal parts. To breathe all night or 2/3 hours daily
  . Harmony is the ideal composition for diffusers and for yoga, meditation, creativity : it balances physical, mental and spiritual energies.
In diffusion : HARMONIE
In friction   : HAR

EO of camomile is seldom used alone.
- MASSAGE OIL FOR CHILDREN : 60 ml WGO + 10 drops EO camomile bring relaxing and relaxation to delicate and "allergic" children.

CORIANDER
"E.O. - STIMUMATING TYPE

- Tonic, aphrodisiac, digestive.
- All types of fatigue, dyspepsiae.

DOSAGE
I.U. : 1 drop 3 x/day on hand in water or honey
E.U. : Frictions and diffusion in atmosphere.
Course: I.U. and E.U. for 3 weeks. **PREVENTION:** 1 course 1
or 2 x/year.

SYNERGIES - RECIPES
- DIGESTIVE FRICTION
  See caraway or DIG Friction
- APHRODISIAC TONIC FRICTION
  10 ml coriander + 5 cinnamon + 15 rosemary + 5 clove + 5
  ginger + 15 marjoram or friction APH : a few drops in frictions
  2 x/day on nape, solar plexus and spine.
- COMPOSITIONS FOR DIFFUSER
  .Invigorating: coriander + rosemary +juniper + pine +
                     vervain + eucalyptus.
                     Proportions to your liking.
  .Aphrodisiac: coriander + ylang-ylang + clove + juniper +
                     cedar + nutmeg.
                     Proportions to your liking.

- BATHS
  Stimulating   2 drops coriander + 2 juniper + 2 rosemary
                     in tble sp. of freeze dried or pulverised sea
                     water or white seaweeds.
  . Aphrodisiac   2 drops coriander + 3 rosewood + 1
                     cinnamon in 2 tble sp. of freeze dried or
                     pulverised water or white seaweeds.
- PERFUMES
  EO of coriander enter in small quantities in men's perfumes.
  . coriander + lavender + clove.
  . coriander + mint + origano.

NOTE : EO of coriander is a sexual and intellectual stimulant.

CYPRESS
"E.O. - CIRCULATION TYPE"

- **Alleviates menopausal circulation (venous)**
- heavy legs, emorrhoids, varicose veins, circulatory problems, hot feet.

DOSAGE
I.U. : 1 drop 3 x/day on hand in water or honey. Abstain in evening.
E.U. : Frictions morning and at 5pm on legs and feet.
Course: I.U. + E.U. 3 weeks **PREVENTION:** 1 course 3/4 x/year.

SYNERGIES - RECIPES
- <u>MENOPAUSAL CIRCULATION AND WEAK ARTERIES</u> (problems for males and females)
  I.U.: 1 drop cypress + 2 drops lemon 3 x/day Morning, 10 am, 2pm.

- <u>COMPOSITION FOR "HOT FEET"</u>
  10 ml cypress + 15 sage + 2 drops lemon 3 x/day. As friction morning and evening. Prevents perspiration or 108 friction.

- <u>COMPOSITION FOR HEAVY LEGS</u>
  10 ml cypress 10 am and 5pm + friction solar plexus.

- <u>WET BED</u>
  1 drop cypress 10 am and 5pm + friction solar plexus.

- <u>CELLULITIS</u>
  associate CEL friction + 108 morning and evening, on feet, legs and buttocks
  + I.U. : 1 drops CEL 3 x/day for 1 week. Alternate with 1 drop 108 3 x/day for 6 weeks.

My advice : 1 course EO cypress 1 or 2 x/year for everyone with bilious or sanguine temperament ... is MUCH ADVISED , as precaution against potential circulatory problems.
Add a course of hydrosol of sage!

EUCALYPTUS
"E.O. - RESPIRATORY PROBLEMS TYPE"

- **N°1 pulmonary antiseptic**
- Prevents colds, flu angina, chills, soothes coughs and bronchitis.

DOSAGE

I.E. : 1 to 3 drops 3/day on hand in water or honey.

E.U. : Friction with 10 to 20 drops, on chest or back, 2 x/day or RES friction.
Diffusion in atmosphere.

Course : I.U. + E.U. during crisis. **PREVENTION**: for 3 weeks before winter.

SYNERGIES -RECIPES

- INHALATION
2 drops eucalyptus + 2 pine + 1 thyme + 5 lavender.
3 to 7 minutes inhalation, 2, 3 x/day.

- BATHS
5 drops eucalyptus + 5 lavender, in 2 tble sp. green seaweeds, powdered
milk or freeze dried or atomised sea water.

- SPECIFIC SYNERGIES FOR I.U. TREATMENT AND FRICTIONS
. Tracheitis   Eucalyptus + pine
. Sinusitis   Eucalyptus + lavender + camomile
. Asthma: Eucalyptus + hyssop
. Bronchitis   Eucalyptus + niaouli + cajeput
. Colds   RES friction (all respiratory problems).

My advice : As soon as you feel a chill, switch on your aroma diffuser, put yourself on a diet for 1 day, take a laxative infusion, 1 or 2 inhalations + 2 frictions + "Anti flu" toddies (see: Cinnamon) and rest in warm room
THE NEXT DAY: IT'S ALL OVER!

NOTE: E.O. of eucalyptus is a requisite for your natural home pharmacy.

JUNIPER
"E.O. - RHEUMATIC PROBLEMS TYPE"

- Anti-rheumatic and diuretic.
- All rheumatic problems, water retention and slimming.

DOSAGE
I.U.   :1 to 2 drops 3 x/day in water and honey.
E.U.   : Frictions 2 x/day, Bath 1 x/day.
Course: I.U. +E.U. 3 weeks
PREVENTION AND UPKEEP: 1 course Spring and Autumn.

SYNERGIES - RECIPES

- SLIMMING
   I.U.: 1 drop juniper + geranium + 1 drop lemon 2 x/day in
      water or honey (see: Lemon file).

- PAIN RELIEF FRICTION
   A few drops of juniper + pine + rosemary + turpentine or RHU
   Friction: 1 to 3 x/day.

- SLIMMING FRICTION
   A few drops juniper + birch + cypress + geranium, as friction on
   legs, buttocks, tummy, arms, 2 x/day.

- SLIMMING BATH
   5 drops juniper + 5 geranium + 5 cypress in 2 tble sp green
   seaweeds + 1 tble. sp. freeze dried or atomised sea water.

- WARMING UP MUSCLES
   A few drops juniper + pine + rosemary + turpentine.
   Used BEFORE and AFTER exercising or VIT Friction.

*My advice: Juniper E. O. dissolves uric stones and residues, helps
with the elimination of kidney waste and slimming .. of course.
Hydrosol of juniper can be an additional slimming, hygienic drink.*

LAVENDER
"E.O. - SMALL CUTS AND CIRCULATION TYPE

- **Soothing, spasmodic, healing.**
- Insomnia, spasm, anxiety, migraine, all wounds:cuts, burns, insect bites. razor rash, acne, dermatosis.

DOSAGE

I.U. : 2 to 3 drops , 2 to 3 x/day on hand in water or honey.
E.U. : A few drop diffused, as friction, or applied:
. To soothe children: On back and chest
. For migraine: On temples
. For anxiety   Evening, on chest and back.
Course: I.U. + E.U. 1 to 3 weeks.   **UPKEEP:** 1 week/month or
                                          3 weeks every 3 months.

SYNERGIES - RECIPES

- INSOMNIA
  I.U.: lavender; marjoram, basil, / 1 drop each at 5pm and before going to bed in water or honey.

- ANXIETY
  E.U.: lavender friction + marjoram: on chest, back and feet each evening. Bath: lavender: each evening (3 to 5 drops)

- RESPIRATORY PROBLEMS
  I.U.: lavender + pine + eucalyptus: 1 drop of each 2 x/day.

- CHILDREN'S INSOMNIA
  I.U.: lavender + orange, 1 drop each 2 x/day in water/honey.

- MIGRAINE
  Friction 15 drops lavender and 3 mint: on temples, forehead, nape and back: 2/3 x/day.

- RELAXATION
. Friction lavender + marjoram + rosewood + petit grain + lemongrass: a few drops at 5pm and before bedtime or friction NER.
. Baths: in 2 tble sp. powdered milk or green seaweeds:
      . lavender 10 drops. rosewood 5 drops
      . lavender 10 drops. marjoram 5 drops

. lavender 10 drops. orange 10 drops.
. Diffusion in atmosphere: all E.O. quoted under Relaxation,
                                    alone or mixed.

- <u>SKIN COMPOSITION:</u>   applied 2 x/day and/or fumigation.
. Dry skin   :lavender + rosewood + rosemary or rose

. Oily skin   :lavender + sage + sassafras
. Itchy skin   :lavender + geranium and hydrosol of
                         lavender.
. Skin to heal   :lavender + geranium + rosemary

- <u>ALL TYPE OF WOUNDS, BURNS, RAZOR RASH, ACNE, SPOTS,
  HERPES, SCURF, MOUTH ULCER</u> : a few drops on wound.

- <u>TOILET WATER</u>: 30 ml lavender in 250 ml alcohol (70°)

*My advice: lavender is almost a panacea! It replaces alcohol and
iodine, soothes, aseptises and heals for children and adults.
It's the first E.O. in the natural pharmacy !
For babies : hydrosol of lavender is remarkable !*

LEMON
"E.O. - SLIMMING WOMAN TYPE"

- **Reinforces natural immunities, tonic, general depurative and blood thinner.**

- General fatigue, obesity, slimming, arteriosclerosis, wounds, herpes, acne, scurf, mouth ulcers.

DOSAGE
U.I. :1 to 2 drops 3 to 5 x/day on hand with water of honey.
E.U. : 3 to 5 drops on skin 1 to 2 x/day (all wounds, acne)
Course: U.I. 2 x/day for 3 weeks
PREVENTION: 1 course each change of season.

SYNERGIES - RECIPES

- SLIMMING
I.U. : lemon + juniper + geranium 1 drop each 2 x/day in water or honey
+ E.U. = caraway + nutmeg - 5 drops each - as friction AFTER MEALS on abdomen.
+ I.U. = marjoram - 1 drop BEFORE BEDTIME, in water or honey.
+ E.U. = friction with NER composition = lavender + marjoram + rosewood + lemongrass + petit grain, on chest, nape and spine (evening) and MIN friction on "round parts".

- SPRING CURE
I.U. : 2 drops EO lemon 3 x/day +3 lemon JUICE in 2 litres water/day for 3 weeks.

- SKIN CARE
. Seborrhea, oily skins = 2 drops lemon + 2 sassafras + 5 lavender, applied twice a day.
. Regenerative mask (all skins) = 2 drops EO lemon + water in 2 tble sp green mud.

. Toothpaste = 2 drops EO lemon + water + mud. Brush teeth
        and massage gums.
. Oil for brittle nails = 10 drops EO lemon in sm sp. WGO
        Massage twice a week.

- <u>PERFUMES</u>
lemon + vervain or lemon, + geranium or lemon + ylang-ylang
15 ml in 100 ml alcohol 70% + 1 ml clary sage as perfume
"fixateur"

- <u>FRESH DRINKS</u>
lemon + geranium or lemon + cedar or lemon + orange or lemon
+ mint or lemon + rosemary.
. 1 drop each + honey + water + ice cubes. Serve as "long drink".
. 1 drop each + honey + warm water. Serve as "Tea".

- <u>CULINARY THERAPY</u>
1 to 4 drops EO lemon in sorbets, flans, desserts, custards.

*My advice : it is WOMAN'S No.1 EO. Each of us should either as
prevention or maintenance, take a CURE OF LEMON (EO + Juice)
at least 1 x/year and take the habit of using EO in drinksinstead
of cordials.*

MARJORAM
"E.O. - "FOOD FOR NERVOUS CELL" TYPE
FOR ANXIOUS PEOPLE AND ANXIETIES

- **Balances neuro-vegetative nervous system, relaxes.**
- Anxieties, depressive state, insomnia.

DOSAGE
I.U. : 1 to 2 drops 2 x/day on hand in water or honey.
E.U. : Friction: 10 to 20 drops, at 5 pm and evening on chest and back.
Bath: 5 drops in 2 tble sp. powdered milk or green seaweeds.
Course: I.U./E.U. : 3 weeks   **UPKEEP:** 1 to 2 courses/year.

SYNERGIES - RECIPES

- FRICTION
  marjoram + lavender + rosewood + petit grain + lemongrass or NER friction: 2 x/day.

- RELAXING BATH
  5 drops marjoram + 5 lavender in 2 tble sp. powdered milk or green seaweeds.

- COMPOSITION FOR DIFFUSER. SLEEP RELAXATION
  . marjoram + lavender + pine + rosewood + vervain
  . marjoram + lavender + petit grain + neroli
  . marjoram + lavender + pine + vervain+ rosewood + mint.

- FRICTION "MIGRAINE, SPASM"
  A few drops marjoram on painful spot and solar plexus.

- RELAXING DRINK
  at 5 pm and at bedtime 2 drops marjoram in warm water + honey.

My advice : even MORE RESULTS with marjoram + basil in synergy. INTERNAL and EXTERNAL TREATMENT IN ALL CASES OF EXHAUSTION OF NERVOUS SYSTEM.

MINT
"E.O. REFRESHING TYPE"

- **Tonic, digestive and bactericide.**
- General fatigue, impotence, bad breath, intestinal parasites.

DOSAGE
I.U. : 1 drop 1/3 x/day, after meals as digestive, or in morning as tonic in water or honey.
E.U.: no prolonged treatment 3 to 7 days as I.U.
UPKEEP : 1 week every 3 months.

SYNERGIES - RECIPES

- COMPOSITION FOR HOT FEET
  15 ml lavender + 3 mint, a few drops as friction on feet morning and evening or before going dancing.

- SLIMMING COMPOSITION
  Rosemary, birch, cypress, juniper, lavender, pine, mint.
  2 frictions/day on legs, tummy and buttocks.

- BATH
  never any mint baths!

- HYGIENIC DRINK
  hydrosol of mint 5 tble sp/litre of water) is children's and adults' cool drink.

- FEET FRICTION
  with hydrosol of mint: morning and evening and before standing up: relieves - refreshes.

Precautions
  - *Never E.O. of mint straight as friction or in bath water, it would turn you into an "iceberg".*
  - *Evening: E.O. mint is a light aphrodisiac and hinders sleep.*

NUTMEG
"E.O. TONIC TYPE"

- **General cerebral stimulant, digestive, aphrodisiac.**
- Intellectual fatigue, impotence, flatulence.....

DOSAGE
I.U.: 1 to 2 drops after meals (preferably caraway + nutmeg)
E.U.: 10 days as I.U.   **UPKEEP:** 1/2 x/year

SYNERGIES - RECIPES

- <u>STIMULATING AND APHRODISIAC FRICTION</u>
  A few drops nutmeg + rosemary + savory geranium + lavender + coriander + pine, morning and evening, as friction on chest, back, soles of feet or VIT friction.

- <u>DIGESTIVE FRICTION</u>
  Caraway 10 drops + nutmeg 10: as friction on abdomen after meals.

- <u>TONIC BATH FOR NERVOUS SYSTEM</u>
  5 drops nutmeg + 5 lavender + 5 marjoram, in 2 tble sp. freeze dried or atomised sea water.

- <u>PERFUME</u>
  In a foundation, E.O. nutmeg, strengthens and gives a manly strain to a soft, flowery fragrance.

- <u>COOKERY</u>
  1 to 3 drops when serving heavy dishes.

NOTE : E.O. nutmeg and E.O. coriander are "sisters" , tonic, physical, sensual and intellectual.

ORANGE - NEROLI - PETIT GRAIN
"E.O. - SLEEPING TYPE"

- **Nervous sedative No 1.**
- Tranquilizer for children, slightly hypnotic, tonicardiac, bactericide.

DOSAGE

I.U.:   orange: 3 to 5 drops at 5pm and bedtime on hand in water or honey.

petit grain: 1 to 2 drops at 5 pm or at bedtime.

neroli: 1/2 to 1 drop at 5 pm or bedtime.

E.U.:   friction with 15 to 20 drops orange, on chest and back before bedtime.

apply a few drops, morning and evening, on skin to regenerate.

Course: 2 x/day for 1 to 3 weeks.   **UPKEEP:** according to needs.

SYNERGIES -RECIPES.

- SEDATIVE FRICTIONS

    15 ml orange + 2 petit grain + 1 neroli, for adults.

    lavender, marjoram, rosewood, petit grain, lemongrass.

    20 to 30 drops of mixture or NER friction.

- SEDATIVE BATH

    5 drops orange + 2 petit grain + 5 lavender in 2 tble sp. milk or green seaweeds.

- "STRONG" SEDATIVE BATH

    1 drop of neroli + 2 petit grain + 5 marjoram in 2 tble sp. powdered milk or green seaweeds.

- COMPOSITION FOR DIFFUSER

    . lavender + petit grain + pine

    . lavender + petit grain + neroli + marjoram.

- PERFUME

    100 ml alcohol (70°C) + 15 ml petit grain + 1 drop neroli

- COOKERY

    3 to 5 drops orange in flans, desserts or cakes.

NOTE : E.O. orange is obtained by expressing the fresh zest of sweet oranges.

E.O. petit grain is obtained by distilling the leaves of Seville oranges.

E.O. neroli is obtained by distilling the flowers of Seville oranges.

ORIGANO
"E.O. -ANTISEPTIC N°1 IN AROMATOGRAM"

- Antiseptic, tonic for nervous system.
- All infectious problems, fatigue.

DOSAGE
I.U: 1 drop 3 x/day on hand in water of honey.
E.U.: frictions ALWAYS DILUTED in other oils.
Course: 3 x/day for 3 weeks   **PREVENTION:** 1 week every 3
months.

SYNERGIES - RECIPES
- TONIC "ANTI-FLU" TODDY
   1 drop origano +1 thyme + 1 cinnamon + 1 clove + 1 geranium
   + 1 ginger (optional) in lemon juice + honey + warm water.

- "INDIGESTION" DRINK
   1 drop origano + 1 clove + 1 ginger + 1 honey + warm water
   AFTER meals

- "TONIC" FRICTION, FLU, CHILLS, FATIGUE
   5 ml origano + 5 marjoram + 5 vervain + 5 basil + 5 lavender
   a few drops 2 x/day on chest : back, soles of feet.

- "ANTI-CELLULIT" FRICTION
   A few drops origano + birch + rosemary + cypress + geranium
   + lavender + pine +mint. Morning and evening on legs,
   buttocks, tummy or CEL friction + 108.

- DISINFECTING COMPOSITION FOR ATMOSPHERE
   15 ml origano + 30 ml lavender + 30 ml geranium + 20 ml
   vervain + 5 ml neroli or cinnamon or sandal wood.

- COMPOSITION FOR BURNS, SEPTIC WOUNDS
   6 ml origano + 8 lavender + 6 geranium.
   A few drops on skin every 3 hours or as compress.

NOTE : • *E.O. origano: no 1 in aromatogram*
         • *Hydrosol of origano offers all the tonic and anti-fatigue*
           properties as daily drink.

PINE
"E.O. - COUGH TYPE

- **Antiseptic for respiratory tracks.**
- Respiratory tracks complaints (colds, tracheitis, pneumonia, asthma, flu..)

DOSAGE
I.U.:　1 to 3 drops 3 x/day on hand in water or honey
E.U.:　friction and 20 to 30 drops pine E. O. in bowl of warm water to inhale 3 to 5 minutes.
Course: 2 x/day for 3 weeks　　**PREVENTION:** 1 course before winter.

SYNERGIES - RECIPES

- "ANTI-COUGH" TODDY
　1 drop pine + 1 eucalyptus + 1 orange + 1 lemon juice + very hot water + honey 2/3 x/day if necessary.

- SOOTHING COUGH FRICTIONS
　. pine / eucalyptus + origano + lavender, a few drops of each;
　. pine + eucalyptus : a few drops of each.

- SCABS
　Apply: 15 ml lavender + 5 pine + 5 eucalyptus + 5 sage 2 x/day.

- HYGIENIC DRINK FOR CHILDREN : soothing
　1 sm. sp. hydrosol of pine in 1 cup of warm water + honey or 1 tble sp./ litre cold water + honey or fructose.

- INFANTS' FRICTION (chills)
　Hydrosol of pine on chest and back, together with hydrosol of lavender (for very young babies).

ROSE/ROSEWOOD
"E.O. - TYPE OF SKIN"

- Strong tissue regenerator, firming up.
- Against wrinkle, every dermatosis, and skin fatigue.

DOSAGE
APPLIED: 4 to 5 drops EO rosewood, 1 to 2 x/day on cleansed
skin as treatment for 3 to 6 weeks.

BATHS: 10 drops in 2 tble sp powdered milks or green
seaweeds to be mixed in bath water.

Course: 6 weeks   **PREVENTION:** 3 to 4 x/year for 3 weeks.

SYNERGIES - RECIPES
- SPECIAL "ANTI-WRINKLE" BODY OIL
  100 ml WGO + 15 rosewood + 1 rose

- SPECIAL FACE OIL
  80 ml WGO + 20 SJWO + 15 rosewood + 1 rose

- FIRMING UP OIL
  100 ml WGO + 10 rosewood + 10 rosemary

- SOOTHING BATHS (see dosage)
  . 5 drops rosewood + 5 lavender or cedar.

- FUMIGATIONS AFTER MASKS
  . Dry skins: lavender + rosewood + rose geranium
  . Oily skins   lavender + rosewood + lemon
  . Wrinkled skins: rosewood + rosemary + sandalwood
  . Itchy skins: rosewood + lavender + camomile

- SCENTED MILKS "AFTER BATH, AFTER SUN"
  . Geranium : 250 ml of neutral body milk + 5 rosewood +
             10 geranium
  . Rose : 250 ml of neutral body milk + 10 rosewood + 5 drops rose.
- TOILET WATER
  . 250 ml alcohol (70° C) + 15 rosewood + 1 rose
- TOILET PERFUME
  . 100 ml alcohol (70 C) + rosewood + 10 drops rose

*Note: In every case you use Rose EO: mix 10 drops of rosewood
EO with 1 drop of EO: much easier to use.
Remember that EO of Rose is one of the most rejuvenative oils.*

SAGE
"E.O. -GYNECOLOGICAL PROBLEMS"

- Anti-perspiration, hypotensive, anti-lacteal.
- General, menopausal fatigue, prevents hot flushes, regulator of menstruation, eliminates excessive perspiration (armpits, feet) hair care, seborrhea, itching, falls ... dries up lactation.

DOSAGE
I.U.: 1 drop 1 to 3 x/day OUTSIDE MEALS on hand in water or honey
E.U.: friction feet 2 x/day.
Course: 1 drop 2 x/day for 1 week   **UPKEEP:** 1 course every
3 months

SYNERGIES -RECIPES
- FRICTIONS, MASSAGES
. Feet: 15 ml sage + 10 lavender, 2 x/day on feet
. Hot feet: 15 ML sage + 10 cypress + 10 lavender + 1 mint.
2 x/day.

- HAIR CARE
10 ml sage + 15 lavender + 5 thyme. 100 drops on scalp 1 x/week, on eve of shampoo for 6 weeks. Eliminates seborrhea, itching ... helps with regrowth, beautifies tired hair.

- SUPER REVITALISING FORMULA
15 ml sage + 15 cedar + 15 lavender + 5 thyme + 1 ylang-ylang.
100 drops 2 x/week or 50 drops 2 x/week, then 1 x/month.
On eve, massage scalp. Keep all night.

- "HEAVY" CONGESTED LEGS FORMULA
15 ml sage + 15 cypress + 3 mint. 30 to 40 drops 2 x/day from ankle to knee + rotating exercises ankles + sleep with propped up legs (10 to 15 cms)

- WARM SPRAYING AFTER FACE CARE
5 drops sage + 5 juniper + 5 lavender. Asepsises and softens.

- BATHS
. Anti-rheumatic: 3 drops sage + 3 lavender + marjoram in
2 tble sp. atomised or freeze dried sea water.
. Heavy legs: 5 drops sage + 5 cypress + 10 lavender in
2 tble sp. green seaweeds

- PERFUMES
In the composition of all perfumes and toilet waters, add a few drops of E.O. clary sage as "fixative" to perfume.

64 sage

SASSAFRAS
"E.O. ANTI-TOBACCO"

- Sudorific, pain killer, skin disinfectant, diuretic
- Tobacco antidote, skin care for acne, ordinary stings or poisonous bites...

DOSAGE
I.U.: 1 to 3 drops 3 x/day in water or honey
E.U. a few drops, morning and evening, applied to skin to regenerate or disinfect.
8 to 10 drops EVERY TWO HOURS, on stings and venom.

SYNERGIES - RECIPES

- ANTI TOBACCO COCKTAIL
1 drop sassafras + 1 sage + 1 geranium + 1 marjoram + 1 lavender + hot water + honey + 1 hydrosol or mint cordial. Serve with ice.

- VERY EFFICIENT ANTI TOBACCO TREATMENT
. 2 to 4 cocktails "anti tobacco" daily
. 2 frictions /day of SAME MIXTURE on solar plexus, back, nape, spine and sole of feet.
. diffusion in atmosphere of mixture vervain + geranium + pine + cedar +mint in equal parts to breathe ALL NIGHT or at least 3 hours/day.

- FUMIGATIONS
2 to 3 drops sassafras + juniper + turpentine, 1 x/day and before care of "loaded" skins.

- MASK
3 drops sassafras + 6 lavender in 2 sm. sp. non-heated honey. Apply for 5 to 8 minutes. Remove with warm water.

- DISINFECTING COMPOSITION FOR SKIN
15 ml sassafras + 15 carrot + 15 lavender, applied morning and evening, 5 to 7 drops alternatively with 15 ml rosewood and 10 drops for skins to be regenerated .. + spraying with hydrosol of cedar.

VERVAIN
"E.O. RELAXATION AND HAPPINESS TYPE"

- **Regulates neuro-vegatative system, tonifies heart, renders harmonious and creative.**
- Fatigue, neuro-vegetative dystonia, anti-dote for snakes' venom.

DOSAGE
I.U.:   1 to 2 drops 2/3 x/day on hand or honey.
E.U.:   10 to 20 drops of vervain : always diluted.
NO FRICTION, NO BATH with UNDILUTED EO EXOTIC VERVAIN.

Diffusion in atmosphere: the E.O. everyone loves, under any circumstance: EXOTIC VERVAIN.

Course: 2 x/day for 3 weeks   **UPKEEP :** 1 week/month or every 3 months.

SYNERGIES - RECIPES

- <u>MORNING TONIC FRICTION:</u>
   5 ml vervain + 5 geranium + 5 lemon, a few drops in morning after cool shower, on chest, solar plexus, nape, back and sole of feet.

- <u>EVENING REGENERATIVE FRICTION</u>
   5 ml vervain + 5 lavender + 5 marjoram + 5 lemongrass, a few drops after hot bath or before bedtime.

- <u>DIFFUSION IN ATMOSPHERE</u>
   . Pleasant: vervain +lemongrass
   . Good temper: vervain + rosewood
   . Anti tobacco: vervain + geranium
   . Ideal: vervain + exotic vervain.

The vervain infusion helps with lactation and childbirth. To take as TREATMENT at the END OF PREGNANCY.

NOTE: I.U. and friction: medicinal vervain.
  Diffusion: exotic vervain; mixture of 3 vervains.
  "My own happy E.O" = my E. O. of "bonheur"

personal notes

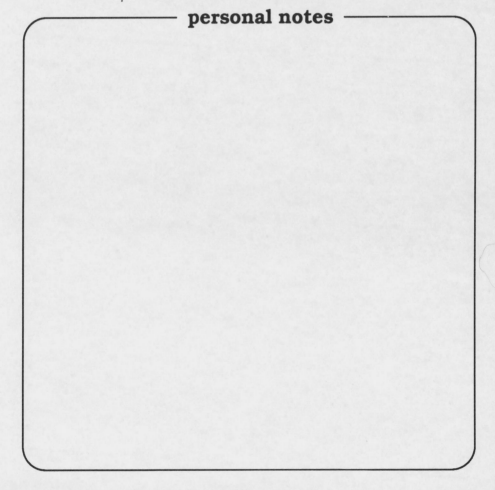

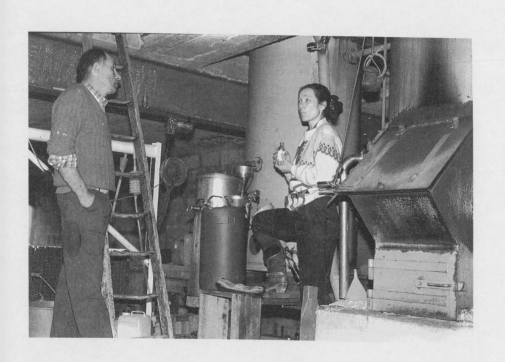

nelly grosjean choosing essences with her private distiller.

CHAPTER 2
THERAPY - Charts and Classifications

- Main problems you may come across.

- Main properties.

- Compose your own natural pharmacy.

- Summary chart.

- Classification by illness.

- Classification by plants.

MAIN PROBLEMS YOU MAY COME ACROSS.

How would you keep standing up if an invisible hand did not support you.
The Koran

DIGESTIVE SYSTEM

Flatulence	Caraway + nutmeg and DIG friction*
Colitis	Cinnamon + DIG friction
Constipation	No E.O.:fresh vegetable juice course + food complements.

Additional advice:
- eat fruit outside meals
- avoid bad food associations
- masticate and take time to eat quietly
- watch for good intestinal elimination.
- + laxative infusion + eat cooked vegetables, toasted bran or wholemeal bread.
- fresh vegetable juice or milk-fermented juices as aperitif.
- a daily hygienic drink with hydrosol of sage, rosemary ....

CIRCULATORY PROBLEMS

Thick blood	Lemon + 108
Heavy legs	Cypress + lemon, CEL friction and 108.
Piles	Cypress + lavender + a treatment of 108.

Additional advice:
- eat raw + spices + garlic, onion ...
- drink a lot outside meals
- exercises

- avoid starch, sugar and animal fat.
- eat less red meat.
- fresh vegetable juice course for 3 weeks before meals
- course of sage, juniper elder......

CELLULITE

Cellulite   Cypress + juniper + lemon (external use)
              Cypress + juniper + birch + turpentine
              or friction CEL + 108 (external use)

Additional advice :
- conscious breathing
- relaxation and sleep
- see "circulatory" advice:
- "cellulite arises from a circulatory problem and a lack of relaxation".

GYNAECOLOGICAL PROBLEMS

Amenorrhea   sage + 108 friction + course of hydrosol of scarified sage.

Dismenorrhea   Same

Painful periods   Same

Leucorrhea   Lavender, vaginal injection.

refer to "Aromatherapie 2, des huiles essentielles pour votre santé", by the same author.

Frictions made by nelly grosjean are by mail-only sale from VIE AROME. See address on last pages

Additional advice
- Strengthening of the abdomen (breathing exercises).
- Regulate food patterns.
- Sexual harmony and mental equilibrium.
- Demystification of psychological disorders which generally occur around menstruation.
- Necessity to discover the causes of disturbance, cleaning out of the body...
- Course of hydrosol of sage, pine or origano.

RHUMATISM

Osteoarthritis
Arthritis   Juniper external + friction against pain RHU.

Additional advice
- Cut down or avoid totally animal proteins during treatment (cheese especially).
- Drink large amounts of water or diuretic infusion (birch, meadowsweet, horsetail...)
- Course of hydrosol of fennel, pine, thyme, celery, juniper, elder).

RESPIRATORY PROBLEMS

Cold, Flu   Eucalyptus + diffusion with Respiratory + RES friction + hydrosol of pine, thyme, hyssop, eucalpytus.

Additional advice
- Breathing exercises.
- Expand your rib cage.
- Control your breathing.
- Clean air and exercises.

- Diet: cut out sweets and starches.
- Importance of nasal hygiene (Works by L. and B. Bardo)

NERVOUS SYSTEM

Insomnia   Marjoram + lavender or orange.
             + diffused lavender.
             + relaxing bath with ABO relax.
             + relaxation friction NER.

Anxiety   Marjoram + basil: nutrition of the nervous cell
             + exotic vervain (diffused)
             + NER or HAR friction.

Tiredness   Rosemary + savory(internal)
             + VIT friction + diffused tonic.

Lack of energy   Morning friction VIT or APH
(sexual, mental,physical)   + rosemary (internal) + hydrosol
                            of rosemary, savory, origano......

Additional advice:
- Cooked or raw food + trace elements + mineral salts (multi-minerals and specialities) + wheat germ oil.
- Importance of good breathing (EO diffusion + ionization).
- Importance of aware relaxation.
- Physical exercises and clean air + relaxation.
- Cut out all stimulants (tobacco, alcohol, coffee, sugar, tea) *The nervous system consumes 14 times more oxygen than any other living cell.*
- Balanced nutrition + super food.
- Recover through sleep (hours before midnight count double).
- Course of hydrosol of marjoram, origano, savory, rosemary alternately.

SKIN   *"Skin, mirror of you health", (Dr. Ribollet)*

Dry skin   Rose + rosewood +hydrosol of rosemary and lavender and sclarified sage.

Wrinkled skin   Rose and rosemary + hydrosol of rosemary and lavender.

Heavy skin   Rose + sassafras + hydrosol of cedar and lavender.

Additional advice
- Draining of liver and intestinal elimination.
- Add of course of B group vitamins (Philaromal from Dietroma).
- Course of wheat germ oil (1sm. sp./day), vitamin A.
- Specific treatment with ABO.
- Regular spraying with hydrosols of rose, sage, lavender, rosemary, cedar.

HAIR

All problems   Sage + thyme + lavender or 106 friction + lotion of hydrosol of wild sage, cedar, thyme, lavender.

Additional advice:
- Freeze-dried yeast (Philaromal).
- Draining of liver (Horseradish).
- Specific teatment (Aromatherapy, beauty).
- The "rawest" nutrition.

SEXUAL PROBLEMS

Tonus   (See tiredness)

Frigidity/Impotence   +general cleansing necessary and
                         personal compositions of
                         revitalisation or APH friction +
                         hydrosol of savory and origano.

Additional advice

- Important to understand simply a harmonious sexual life.

- Exercises and fresh air.

- Balanced nutrition (+ vegetable juices + food complements).

- Loosening and relaxing.

- In all cases, add these additional advices to recommendations for a good, hygienic lifestyle.

TABLE
ESSENTIAL OILS: MAIN PROPERTIES

MAIN PROPERTIES	CORRESPONDING ESSENTIAL OILS
Slimmers	**Lemon, Juniper, Rose, Geranium,** Birch (see Juniper for baths and slimming frictions).
Pain Killers	**Lavender, Majoram, Camomile. Clove** (teeth). Cajeput See Juniper.
Antibiotics	**Origano** No 1 from Aromatogram. **Cinnamon. Thyme. Clove. Savory** Cajeput Pine. Lavender.
Anti-wrinkles	**Rose. Rosewood. Rosemary.** Sandal. Ylang-Ylang.
Antiseptics	
- Intestinal	**Caraway. Cinnamon.** Eucalyptus **Thyme.** Bergamot. Origano. Nutmeg.
- Genito-urinary	**Sandalwood. Ylang-Ylang.** Cedar. Hyssop.
- Pulmonary /Respiratory	**Cajeput. Thyme. Origano.** Niaouli. Pine. Rosemary.
Anti-spasmodics	**Camomile.** Bergamot. Tarragon. Basilic.
Anti - perspiration	**Sage**
Anti-tobacco	**Sassafras.** Rose geranium. Marjoram. Lavender.
Aphrodisiacs	**Cinnamon. Ginger. Rosemary. Savory. Ylang- Ylang.** Nutmeg. Coriander. Sandal. Clove. Rosewood. Ginger recipes.

In bold : essential oils to be favoured for their required specific property.

Soothin	See pain killers
- Pains	**Lavender, Marjoram, Neroli.** Orange, Petit Grain.
- Relaxation	**Marjoram. Lavender.** Camomile.
- Anti-depressing	**Basilic + Marjoram.** Vervain
Scar healers	**Lavender, Rose geranium. Rosemary.** Rosewood. Sandalwood.
Digestive	**Caraway. Nutmeg. Coriander. Cumin Mint.** Tarragon. Basilic. Rosemary.
Diuretic	**Lemon. Birch. Juniper.** Sandalwood. Cedar.
Respiratory	**Eucalyptus. Pine. Thyme. Hyssop.** Cajeput. Niaouli.
Revitalising	
- Intellect	**Coriander.** Tarragon. Clove. Rosemary. See & Rosemary.
- Glandular system	**Sandalwood. Savory. Ylang-Ylang. Rosemary. Cinnamon.**
- General state	**Rosemary. Savory. Origano.** Coriander.
- Sexual function	See Aphrodisiacs.
- Nervous system	**Basilic + Majoram.** Vervain.
Essential oil from the aromatogram	**Origano. Savory. Cinnamon. Thyme.** Clove. Cajeput. Pine. Lavender

In bold: essential oils to be favoured for their required specific property.

The Almighty gave the earth medicines
and the wise man will not ignore them.
The Ecclesiast.

COMPOSE YOUR OWN "NATURAL PHARMACY".

Green Clay (tube)
Any wound, sting, cut, scratch ... brings out foreign bodies, splinter, pus .....heals scar tissue.

Chloride of magnesium
Any affectation, prepare 1 litre of water with 20 grams of chloride of magnesium. take 2 lge sp./2xday. or every 3 hours.

Essential Oils Lavender + Rose Geranium: heal, soothe.
On all wounds, sting, burn, small cut, razor rash, cut ... Can be used in alternatively with clay poultices.

Essential Oil Mint: Digestive, refreshing.
1/2 drops after meals

Essential oils caraway + nutmeg : strong digestive (or DIG friction) 2 or 3 drops after meals + 20 drops friction on abdomen, after meals, in case of wind, flatulence...

Essential Oil Lemon: General Antiseptic.
2/3 drops applied on breaking spots, herpes, impetigo several times a day.

Essential Oil Sage: Anti-perspiration .A few drops applied on armpits and feet avoid unpleasant perspiration (fr. 108)
1 drop in water or honey 3 x/day to facilitate painful menstruation + CEL friction at the base of tummy.

Essential Oils Rosemary or Origano or Thyme: powerful antibiotic and antiseptic.
A drop (whichever) 3 to 5 times/day in case of biological disorders or viral or microbial origins (angina, asthma, hepatitis, chills....)

Essential Oil Eucalyptus: pulmonary and respiratory antiseptic.

1/3 drops, 3 x/day + friction chest and back + aroma diffusion: avoid flu ....

RES friction efficiently allows friction and diffusion.

Essential Oils Juniper + Pine + Rosemary + Turpentine or RHU friction.

Instantly soothe any pain be they:rhumatism, arthritis, osteoarthritis, muscles ... also warms up before any exercise.

Essential Oil Cinnamon: intestinal antiseptic.

1 drop, 2, 3 x every 2 hours, stops diarrhea in less than 4 hours.

Essential Oil Camomile: antispasmodic

1 to 2 drops 3x/day + friction on temples and around nose, calms sinusitis.

Essential Oils Marjoram + Lavender or NER friction: calming, relaxing.

Few drops as friction on temples and base of neck stop all headaches .... and help sleep.

Essential Oil Orange or Lavender: sedative for children.

1 drop Orange on 1 sm. sp of honey before going to bed + friction on chest and back with Orange + Lavender, makes children sleep.

Oil of St. John's wort - Our grandmother's "red oil": on sunburns, burns: soothes and heals.

To be applied on neck and spine, according to Dr. Breuss, a German doctor from early this century who used to treat with oil of St. John's wort and courses of vegetable juices, this oil has the particular effect of ""re-inflating" intervertebral cartilages".

SUMMARY CHART : DIRECTIONS FOR USE
AND GENERAL DOSAGE

Dosage	Use	Treatment	General Use
DIFFUSION	In atmosphere Aroma diffuser.	Daily 1	15ml for one week of diffusion
FRICTIONS	On body	3 weeks to 3 months	20 -50 drops/fct 1 to 3 X /day.
INTERNAL USE	Absorption	1 - 3 weeks when necessary	1 - 3 drops 3 x/day
INHALATIONS	Inhalator		3 - 10 drops of inhalator
BATHS	Health baths and showers	Crisis 1 - 2 baths/day 1 bath, 1-3/day	3 - 10 drops/bath
FUMIGATION	Skin	Before care 1 x/week	3 - 10 drops/bowl
MASKS	Skin	1 - 2 x/week	1 - 5 drops mask
MILKS	Skin and body	daily	15 ml in 250 ml/milk
BEAUTY FRICTIONS	Skin	3 weeks 2 x/day	3 - 5 drops frct.
FOOT	Feet	Daily 1 - 2 frictions	10 - 20 drops frct.
HAIR FRICTIONS	Hair	6 weeks	50 - 100 drops frct
OILS MASSAGES	Body	Daily	15 - 30 ml in 100ml oil
BEAUTY OILS	Face	From 3 weeks 3 - 4 x/year	5 - 15ml of special oil anti-wrinkle
PERFUME	Perfume Toilet water		15 ml in 100 ml alc 70°C 15 ml in 250 ml alc 70°C

Precautions: please refer to recipes given in various files on essential oils.
Abbreviations: frct- friction x/ - multiply day/month alc - alcohol.

CLASSIFICATION PER ILLNESS

Illness	Corresponding essential oils
Acne	LEMON, SASSAFRAS. Eucalyptus see Skin & Cajeput oil
Acne rosacea	CYPRESS. ROSEWOOD.
Allergy	CAMOMILE. Cedar. Rosewood. Lavender. Diffusion in atmosphere.
Alopecia	see Hair
Amenorrhea	PARSLEY, LEMON, NUTMEG, Cypress, Sage, Geranium.
Angina	LEMON. SAVORY.ORIGANO. rose geranium. Camomile.
Anguish,Anxiety	BASILIC + MARJORAM see anti-depressive and Lavender
Anti-wrinkle	ROSE, ROSEWOOD. ROSEMARY.
Armpits	see anti-perspiration
Asthma	HYSSOP. Lavender. Camomile. Cajeput oil. Eucalyptus
Bandages	Clay powder + LAVENDER + ROSEMARY + ROSE GERANIUM
Biliary lithiasis	see Gallstones
Blisters	LAVENDER
Boils	LAVENDER +LEMON
Breath (fetid)	MINT. Nutmeg
Breasts(chapped)	see chaps.
Bronchitis	HYSSOP. NIAOULI. CAJEPUT OIL see respiratory E.O.
Burns	LAVENDER + ROSE GERANIUM. Niaouli
Cancer (prevention)	ONION. ROSE.
Cellulite	BIRCH. JUNIPER. CYPRESS; Origano. Lavender. Rosemary
Chaps	Lemon juice + LAVENDER.
Chilblains	LAVENDER + Lemon juice.
Childbirth (to help)	vervain infusion + SAGE essential oil.
Cholera	MINT. ORIGANO. THYME.
Cholesterol(excess)	ROSEMARY + ROSE GERANIUM.
Circulation	LEMON. CYPRESS. SAGE see circulatory E.O.
Cirrhosis	ORIGANO. ROSEMARY.
Cold	
- Simple cold	all essential oils in the aromatogram.

- Hay fever	Camomile. Lavender. Hyssop.
Colonbacillosis	ORIGANO. Origano. No. 1 in aromatogram.
Colic	CINNAMON. Caraway.
Conjunctivie	juice of lemon. see recipe Lemon
Constipation	plants, a balanced diet, but no specific essential oil for constipation.
Corpulence	see Slimmers
Cough - Tracheitis	PINE + EUCALYPTUS + coated pills (clay)
Crevices	LAVENDER. + LEMON. rosewood
Cuts	LAVENDER. see wounds.
Cystitis	CAJEPUT OIL. SANDALWOOD. Lavender.
Dental abcess	CLOVE, see Teeth.
Dental cavities	CLOVE, Lavender.
Dental (pains)	Children: CAMOMILE.
Dermatitis	see Skin E.O.
Diabetes	JUNIPER. EUCALYPTUS; LEMON. + Robert Geranium (plant)
Diarrhea/Dysentery	CINNAMON. Caraway.
Digestion	see Digestive E.O.
Distending	see Flatulence, digestive.
Dysmenorrhea	SAGE. CYPRESS. Tarragon
Dyspepsia	see Digestive
Emopytysis	LEMON. EUCALYPTUS, CAMOMILE.
Enterocolitis	LAVENDER. CARAWAY. Camomile.
Epidemics (prevention)	see Antiseptics, Antibiotics, (mainly diffused in the atmosphere.
Excitement	see Soothers;
Eczema	ROSE. Lavender. Rose Geranium. Juniper. Sandalwood.
Fatigue	fatigue or the exhaustion of vital energies necessitates a re-shaping of life hygiene: balanced diet, exercises, breathing, fresh air, relaxation, positive thinking, harmony.
- General	LEMON. ROSE GERANIUM. Rosemary. Origano.
- Physical	ROSEMARY, CORIANDER. Origano.
- Nervous	BASILIC + MARJORAM. Lavender.
- Intellectual	Coriander. Clove. Rosemary. Rosewood + Cinnamon + Camomile + diffusion in the atmosphere

- Sexual	Cinnamon. Ginger. Nutmeg. Coriander. Savory. Rosemary. Sandalwood. Ylang-ylang.
- Moral	<u>Vervain in diffusion or Harmonie.</u> see anti-depressive.
- Muscular	Rosemary + Juniper. Turpentine.
Fevers	LEMON + SAGE
Flatulence	CARAWAY. NUTMEG. Coriander. Cumin.
Flu	EUCALYPTUS. THYME. <u>Origano.</u> CINNAMON. see Cinnamon for anti-flu today
FEET	
- Hot	LAVENDER + MINT + ROSEMARY + Rosewood + Rose Geranium see Cypress recipe.
- Sweaty	SAGE + CYPRESS + LAVENDER
Gonorrhea	Sandalwoo. Thuya. Savory.
Gout	JUNIPER. Cajeput oil. Rosemary.
GUMS	
- To strengthen	LEMON
- Gingivitis	LEMON + <u>powdered clay.</u>
HAIR	
- Loss	LAVENDER + SAGE + THYME.
- Improvement	YLANG-YLANG. CEDAR. Lavender. Sage. Thyme.
- Greasy	LAVENDER + SAGE + THYME + CEDAR.
Headaches	LAVENDER. CAMOMILE.
Head Cold	see Head Cold.
Healing	LAVENDER + ROSE GERANIUM. Rosemary. Niaouli.
Heart Palpitations	PETIT GRAIN. NEROLI. Mint.
Herpes	LEMON. ROSE GERANIUM. ORIGANO.
Hiccup	TARRAGON.
Hypertension	HYSSOP.
Hypotension	ROSEMARY
Hysteria	NEROLI. Lavender. Majoram.
Heavy Legs	CYPRESS + SAGE+ Mint + Rose Geranium (external)
Impotence	see Aphrodisiacs.
Indigestion	see Digestions & Clove recipe.
Infections	see Antiseptics E.O.
Insect Bites	LAVENDER + GERANIUM + CINNAMON. see Cinnamon recipe.

INSOMNIA
- Children   LAVENDER. ORANGE.
- Adults   LAVENDER.MARJORAM. Petit Grain.
                                Neroli. Orange.
Intestinal ferments   see Digestive and intestinal Antiseptics.
                                CARAWAY "No 1 intestinal oxygeniser."
Irritability   BASILIC + MARJORAM. NEROLI +
                                ORANGE. LAVENDER.
Jaundice   ORIGANO. ROSEMARY. LEMON.
Laryngitis   LAVENDER + PINE + CAJEPUT OIL.
                                see Respiratory E.O.
Leucorrhea   SANDALWOOD + LAVENDER. Juniper.
                                Hyssop.
Lice   GERANIUM; Lavender. Sage.
Liver (deficiency)   ROSEMARY. MINT.
Longevity   hygienic diet, exercises, *breathing and
                                regular use of essential oils* as frictions
                                and diffusion and positive thinking are all
                                factors for good health and longevity.
Loss of strength   see Fatigue
Malaria   ORIGANO. THYME. CINNAMON. SAVORY.
                                and essential oils from the aromatogram.
Melancholia   see Revitalizers.
Menopause (troubles)   SAGE. cypress. Lemon.
Migraine   LAVENDER. CAMOMILE. MINT.
                                Marjoram. see Lavender recipe.
Medical Intoxication   MINT
Menstruation and
female problems   see Amenorrhea. Dysmenorrhea.
                                Leucorrhea.
Mouth Ulcer   Lemon.
Mumps   CAMOMILE (external). Lemon Juice.
                                see Lemon recipe.
Muscles   ROSEWOOD. LAVENDER. SAGE. Savory.
Mycoses (feet)   LAVENDER + SAGE + ROSE.
Nausea   ROSEMARY. TARRAGON. MINT.
                                see Clove recipe.
Nephritis   SANDAL. YLANG-YLANG. JUNIPER.
Nervous breakdown   BASILIC + MARJORAM.
                                see Anti-depressive E.O.
Neurasthenia   see Anti-depressive E.O.
Nicotine addiction   SASSAFRAS; Rose Geranium. Marjoram.
Nocturnal perspiration   SAGE

Obesity	JUNIPER. LEMON. see Slimmers. Recipe: Lemon or Juniper.or Rose Geranium.
Osteoarthritis	see Anti-rhumatism E.O.
Otitis	Juice of Lemon. see Lemon recipe.
Overwork	see Revitalizers.
Oxyuris	GARLIC (essential oil diluted 2%) ORIGANO. CARAWAY. MINT.
Pains	see Pain killers.
Papillome	THUYA (external).
Paralysis (after effects)	ALL ESSENTIAL OILS in friction or in diffusion in the atmosphere to regenerate the whole body.
PERSPIRATION	
- Excessive	SAGE + CYPRESS + LAVENDER + ROSEWOOD. + MINT.
- Feet	SAGE. CYPRESS. LAVENDER. see Hot Feet.
Piles	LAVENDER + CYPRESS (external).
Pneumonia	see Respiratory E.O.
Prostate	THUYA. SANDAL.
Pruritis	LAVENDER.
Psoriasis	see Cajeput oil recipe.
Psychic instability	BASILIC + MARJORAM. BERGAMOT.
Rhinitis	LAVENDER. CAMOMILE
Rhumatism	JUNIPER + Pine + Turpentine + Rosemary. + Eucalyptus.
Seasickness	MINT
Scabies	see Pine.
Scabs	see Lavender recipe.
Scurf	LEMON. Rose Geranium.
Seborrhea	
- Skin	LAVENDER + SAGE + ROSEWOOD
- Hair	LAVENDER + SAGE + THYME + YLANG- YLANG. see Sage recipe.
Senescence	LEMON. see Longevity.
Sinusitis	CAMOMILE. Lavender. Lemongrass. Eucalyptus.
Sciatica	Lavender + Marjoram + Lemongrass (external)
Shingles	see Rose geranium recipe.

SKIN	
- Care	CARROT. ROSEWOOD. LEMON. ROSE.
- Cleansing	SASSAFRAS. CEDAR. Juniper. Cajeput.
- Revitaliser	ROSEMARY. ROSEWOOD. SANDAL WOOD. ROSE. Ylang-Ylang.
- Anti-wrinkle	ROSEWOOD + ROSE.
- Dermatoses	LEMON. LAVENDER. see Lavender recipe.
Slimming	see Slimmers.
Smell, loss of	All essential oils diffused in the atmosphere. Basic leaves
Sores	
- Infected	LAVENDER. CAJEPUT oil.
- To heal	LAVENDER. ROSE GERANIUM. ROSEMARY. Niaouli. Hyssop.
Spasms	see Anti-spasmodics.
Stiffness	ROSEMARY. Turpentine.
Stiff neck	LAVENDER + MARJORAM +LEMONGRASS. see Pain killers.
STONES	
- Urinary	JUNIPER. Sandal. Ylang-Ylang. Lemon.
- Bile	JUNIPER. SANDAL. LEMON. Rosemary.
Sprains (ankle)	ROSEMARY. Juniper + clay poultice.
Sunstroke	LAVENDER. GERANIUM.
Teeth (infection)	CLOVE. see Clove recipe.
Tetanus	see Antiseptics.
Thrush (candida albicans)	ORIGANO. THYME. Cinnamon. Savory. Clove.
Tuberculosis	CAJEPUT OIL. PINE. THYME. ORIGANO.
ULCER	
- Stomach	LAVENDER. Raw potato juice.
- Varicose	see Circulatory and Antiseptics.
Varicose	CYPRESS. LEMON.
Vertigo	CAMOMILE. MINT. LAVENDER.
Vulvitis/ vulvo-vaginitis	LAVENDER (external).
Warts	THUYA
Weight Loss	see Slimmers.
Whitlow	LAVENDER (external) see Antiseptics
WOUNDS	LAVENDER

PLANTS - CLASSIFICATIONS

Common name	Primary Action	Complementary Action	E.O. "type"
BASILIC	Tonic	Antispasmodic	....
BERGAMOT	Intestinal infections	Dermatoses	....
CAJEPUT OIL	Chronic lung	Anti-neuralgic infections	....
CAMOMILE	Antispasmodic	Softener	Sinusitis
CARAWAY	Dyspepsies	oxygenizer	Flatulence
CEDARWOOD	Dematoses	Genito-urinary	....
CINNAMON	Tonic antiseptic	Sexual tonic	Diarrhea
CITRONELLA	Removes mosquitoes	....	....
CORIANDER	General stimulant	....	....
CLOVE	Anaesthetic toothache Stimulant Memory	Antiseptic	Toothache memory
CYPRESS	Circulatory problems	Deep and Superficial Cellulite Acne rosacea	Circulation
EUCALYPTUS	Sterilises	Fluidifies pulmonary mucosities	Respiratory
JUNIPER	Diuretic anti-rhumatism	Slimmer	Rhumatism
GINGER	Stimulates glandular functions	Ovaries Testicles	"Aphrodisiac"
HYSSOP	Chronic pulmonary complaints	Healer external use	Asthma

LAVENDER	Soothing cutaneous pulmonary Healer	Regulator of nervous system	Small sores relaxing.
LEMON	General Depurative	Increase Immunities	Women
LEMONGRASS	Tropical Antiseptic	....	....
MARJORAM	Anxieties Anguish Insomnia Depressions	Soother Regenerator	"Food for nervous cell"
MINT	General and digestive Stimulant	Refreshing	....
NUTMEG	General and cerebral stimulant	Excites the brain and the senses. Digestive	Tonic
NEROLI	Nervous sedative	Cellular revitaliser	Sleep
NIAOULI	Pulmonary Antiseptic	....	....
ORANGE	Nervous sedative	Tranquillizer children.	Sleep
ORIGANO	No. 1 Antiseptic in aromatogram	General stimulating	Antibiotic
PETIT GRAIN	Nervous sedative	Tranquillizer	Sleep
PINE	Pulmonary Antiseptic	Expectorating	Cough
ROSEMARY	Digestive and heart tonic	Liver tonic	Tonus for sportsmen.
ROSE	Anti-cancer	Tissue Re-juvenator	No I anti-wrinkle
ROSE GERANIUM	Energizes cortical-suprarenal	Healer	"Sweet tooth"

ROSEWOOD	Tissue regenerator	Toner	Skin
SAGE	Diuretic Ovaries regulator	Anti-sweat	Gynecological
SANDALWOOD	Genito-urinary antiseptic	Aphrodisiac Skin care	....
SASSAFRAS	Tobacco antidote	....	Anti-tobacco
SAVORY	Genital and intellectual stimulant	Stimulates nutrition	Sexual and physical tonic
TARRAGON	Diuretic and Ovaries regulator	Anti-Sweat	Gynecological
TURPENTINE	Diuretic	Anti-rhumatism	Provokes perspiration
THUYA	Genito-urinary Antiseptic	Worts	Prostatitis
THYME	Powerful Antiseptic	Stimulant	No.2 antibiotic
VERVAIN	Favours Harmony	Arouses creativity	Happiness
YLANG-YLANG	Sexual Stimulant	Antiseptic	....

Essential oils "type" in bold and correspond to my own designation.
Essential Oils "type": please note that in all cases for some persons the essential oil "type" will bring a positive result for any given indication.

Just as " major essential oils from the aromatogram" exist the same applies to the essential oils "type".

For example: Caraway, the essential oil "type" for flatulence is also, in all circumstances, the best essential oil for this ailment;

.... : no essential oil "type".

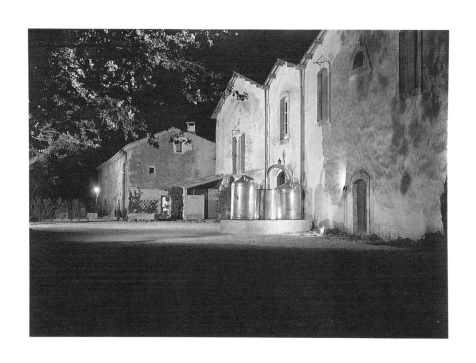

La Chevêche en Provence
Information centre on Holistic Medicine.

CHAPTER 3

ESSENTIAL OILS FOR BEAUTY

- **the beauty pharmacy**

- **prepare our own beauty products**
    - **aromatic bath**
    - **aromatic oils for the body**
    - **aromatic oils for massage**
    - **aromatic frictions with E.O.**
    - **aromatic oil for the face**
    - **aromatic oil for the hair**
    - **aromatic oil for the feet**
    - **aromatic oil for nails**
    - **fumigations**
    - **masks**
    - **aftershave**
    - **perfumes**
    - **face tonics**

abbreviations	WGO	: wheatgerm oil
	SJWO	: St John's wort oil
	O	: Oil
	ABO	: aromatic oil

The "Beauty" Pharmacy

essential oils	hydrosols	various
rosewood	cornflour	clay(powder/tube)
camomile	camomile	honey
lemon	juniper	seaweeds(powder)
juniper	lavender	chorumagène
rose geranium	rosemary	purgative limonette
lavender	sage	castor oil
rosemary	thyme	san pellegrino magnesia
rose		wheatgerm oil
sandal wood		St John's wort oil.
sassafras		sesame oil
sage		1 mixer
ylang-ylang		some empty bottles (brown glass)

Before mixing your preparations relax, loosen, smile to yourself: it's an enjoyable moment.

Natural aromatic essential oils are fragile and powerful "friends".

Treat them with consideration, respect and love.

Respect Dosage.

Always use coloured glass bottles for your preparations and become ... the perfect " pharmacist-alchemist" of your own beauty.

Prepare your own beauty products
Aromatic Preparations

- bath oils
- body oils/massage oils
- frictions
- face oils/eyes (outline)
- hair/feet/nails/oils
- fumigations/inhalations
- masks
- toilet water/perfumes
- aftershave
- compresses for eye/burns/vaginal injections/enema
- face tonics.

How to take an efficient aromatic bath

Water temperature : 36 to 39 degrees or 40, as you wish.

Duration: 5 to 30 minutes

Frequency: acute illness : 1 to 2 baths/day

chronic illness: 1 bath/day or every other day.

Mandatory rest time after each bath: 5 to 15 minutes.

Aim of bath : to relax, open up pores and eliminate toxins.

- dip into an aromatic bath at pleasant temperature
- relax 5 to 15 minutes in bath, rub with water.
- when getting out add very hot water for 30 seconds then come out.
- do not dry yourself, wrap into a bathrobe.
- lie down with a towel wrapped around you neck, feet and body + 1 rug.
- relax at least 5 to 15 minutes.

Relaxation and hyperemia provoked by the last warm phase of the bath, allow for perspiration and elimination of toxins. The very short period of high hear has not affected either the vascular or cardiac systems.

This bathing formula ensures a maximum of efficiency without any inconvenience.

If the bath is tonic:

after 5 minutes rest take a cool or cold shower, and rub yourself with a composition of tonic or stimulating essential oils.

If the bath is relaxing:

continue this relaxation and why not go to sleep relaxed enjoying this well being all night through.

Bath

All aromatic oils for baths can be used in showers.

In which case, use natural solvents rather than lathers of milks.

Speciality:

ABO or nelly grosjean's precious oils are to be used 5 drops in bath water.

AROMATIC OILS FOR BATHS

Aromatic oils do not mix with water, they have therefore to be mixed with a natural solvent before introducing them to water, otherwise unpleasant burns will occur!

Only E.O. of lavender can be used as such in bath water!

- for small infants:. use hydrosol of lavender 2 tble sp/bath
- for babies: 5 drops of EO lavender in 1 sm sp of WGO or sweet almonds oil or hydrosol.
- for adults 5 to 10 drops of EO lavender or 5 to 10 drops aromatic oil for bath or 1 glass of hydrosol.

HOW TO PREPARE AN OIL FOR YOUR BATH

In general, 10° to 30% of EO are diluted in a natural "solvent"

natural "solvents" : • WGO = wheatgerm oil
- full milk powder
- seaweed powder
- egg yoke shampoo
- neutral foundation.

Aromatic oils for baths: in 60 ml add.

cinnamon: cinnamon 5 ml + cedar 10ml (optional)

hindu: ylang-ylang 15 ml

oriental: sandalwood 5ml + rosewood 5ml or cedar 5ml.

to perspire: turpentine 60 ml (in 60 ml WGO)

tonic: rosemary 15ml

relaxing: marjoram 5ml, lavender 15ml

refreshing after sunburns:lavender 15 ml, mint 5ml or rose geranium 10 ml, mint 5ml.

relieving rose geranium 15 ml

rejuvenating and against dry skin: rosewood 10 ml, rose geranium 5ml, rose 1ml

wood oil to perspire:	rosewood 5ml, cedarwood 5 ml, turpentine 30 ml sandalwood 3 ml.
soothing for children:	lavender 20 ml, orange 5 ml, mandarine 2 ml.
aphrodisiac:	lavender 30 ml, ylang-ylang 10 ml, sandalwood 5 ml, rose 1ml
calming:	camomile 3ml, neroli 1 ml, lavender 20 ml.

All EO can be used in baths, diluted with a natural "solvent" 3 to 10 drops according to EO selected:

for example: marjoram, birch, juniper, rose geranium 5 to 10 drops. neroli, vervain, camomile 1 drop. rose 1/2 drop., turpentine 10 drops.

> **Caution: used straight, not diluted, in bath water, they are liable to "burn".**

Hydrosols for baths :2 tble sp per bath

relaxing	:lavender or camomile
elimination	:juniper
tonic	:savory, rosemary, origano
fresh	:mint
pleasant	:vervain, marjoram
soft	:wild rose, lavender, neroli.

AROMATIC OILS FOR MASSAGES

- aromatic oils for baths and body can by used for massages: they only have to be diluted.
- to different types of massage correspond different oils: "oily", "greasy" or "penetrating".

dosage 3 to 10% of EO in oil for massage

INGREDIENTS

Wheatgerm oil	rich in vitamin E, rejuvenative. penetrates fast without greasing.
coco oil	fat, thick, it remains for a while on the surface.
St John's wort oil	double maceration of flowers in olive oil - 0,5 % acidity - is said to pump up cartilages (Dr Breuss)
sesame oil	light, fine, penetrates and .... "Sesame open up"
sweet almond oil	light, penetrating, becomes rancid fast.

PLEASE NOTE

shiatsu	use EO or oils for bath strongly concentrated (30 to 40%) in EO in WGO.
rolfing-magnetism Californian	apply Natural EO: see - frictions
physiotherapy	use neutral cream, coco oil, olive oil to which are added WGO, SJWO and EO.

1) fatty massage oil
  - select 3 to 5 ml EO or 10ml ABO
    add 120 ml coco oil or coco oil + olive oil in equal parts.

2) rejuvenative and penetrating massage oil
 - select 3 to 5 ml EO or 10ml ABO
   add 60 ml WGO + 30 ml sesame oil + 30 ml SJWO

NOTE: WGO is rich in vitamin E, excellent for skin, toning and nervous system. Dont forget that any bodycare product should be "edible": it is absorbed by the skin and "digested".

3) neutral massage oil
 - select 3 to 5 ml EO or 10ml ABO
   add 100 ml almond oil or basic neutral cream

4) aromatic massage oil for children
 - 3 to 10 ml EO lavender, eucalyptus, orange or camomile or ABO relax.
 - 30 ml WGO, 30 ml sesame, 30 ml sweet almond.

NOTE: Children love orange and camomile! Remember to play with basic oils to obtain the correct fluidity and speed for penetration.

Another option: add the selected EO later.

AROMATIC FRICTIONS WITH EO

Originally, Egyptian perfume was a balm, an ointment, with a flower base of plants prepared by the priest, the physician, the oracle, for the health of body and spirit. Used morning or evening to develop physical or mental faculties, love, trust, creativity or communication, much as the 12 moons, 12 months, 12 zodiac signs, 12 apostles ... 12 little problems of our daily life. Developed over the past 15 years, they correspond to the 12 metabolic functions of our wonderful body.

A friction with EO harmonises, re-balances, tonifies, relaxes and re-assures; it is our protection just as the fragrance of a flower is its protective envelope.

A friction with EO brings a new energy needed by our body continuously drwan to the external agressions. You will appreciate a friction morning or evening, on the solar plexus, nape, spine or sole of your feet.

Protection, harmony, vitality, regeneration.

My 12 "frictions" stock and restore nature's vital elements, an energy useful and necessary to our well being.

Why use essential oil in frictions?

- **We know that, after applying essential oils on the skin, within 4 hours, the essential oils are in our blood and lymph.**
- Furthermore, the elective property of essential oils gives the following advantage:

Essential oils in friction, or on any part of the body, will inevitably be attracted to the weak organ or the disturbed function.

We shall therefore talk of "beauty frictions" those each of us should apply to increase his/her vital potential, favour the body awakening in the morning relaxation and good sleep at night.

- tonic morning frictions, evening relaxing, digestive, respiratory, circulatory, "pain reliever", aphrodisiac.
- frictions for the skin, feet, hair.

When to apply frictions?

Morning, 6am to 12 noon	Morning tonic
Evening, 6pm to midnight	Evening relaxing
5 pm and before bedtime	Aphrodisiac
After the 3 meals	Digestive
Morning and evening	Respiratory
Morning, 5pm and	
before bedtime	Circulatory
Morning and evening	Feet

How to apply frictions?

- 20 drops in the palm of the hand and apply to the parts to be treated and to solar plexus.

Where to apply frictions?

On the whole body:	Tonic
Chest, nape, spine:	Relaxing
Arms, legs, sole of feet:	Aphrodisiac
and solar plexus	
Chest, back and solar plexus	Respiratory
Tummy, abdomen and solar plexus	Digestive
Painful part and solar plexus	Pain relief
Feet, legs and solar plexus	Circulatory
Feet only	Feet
Scalp only	Hair
Face only	Face

How much?

- Body frictions	20 to 30 drops
- Tummy and abdomen frictions	15 to 20 drops
- Pain frictions	5 to 10 drops
- Legs frictions	10 to 20 drops
- Feet frictions	10 drops
- Hair frictions	50 to 100 drops
- Face frictions	5 to 7 drops
Chest and back frictions	20 to 30 drops

For children with delicate skin:

Frictions must always be mixed to an identical volume of wheatgerm, almonds or olive oil.

Never use non-diluted frictions for infants under 6 months old.

Precautions

- The following EO can be used as such and not diluted: rosewood, cajeput, camomile, cedar, lemon, cypress, eucalyptus, juniper, rose-geranium, lavender, marjoram, myrrh, niaouli, orange, petit grain, pine, rosemary, sandalwood, ylang-ylang.

- EO which must be diluted:
applied directly onto the skin they are liablle to burn, chill, or simply be unpleasant!
green anise, basil, bergamot, cinnamon, coriander, tarragon, ginger, clove, lemongrass, mint, nutmeg, neroli, origano, rose, savory, sassafras, sage, turpentine, thuya, thyme, vervain.

How to dilute them

IN EO lavender, WGO or any other basic oil.

see - Body oils, oils for massages.

EO : AROMATIC FRICTIONS
Properties:

APH action	energiser for cortico-adrenal, ideal for fatigue, memory, sexual drive,businessman's stress...
NER relaxation	relaxing of the nervous system, favours refreshing sleep, soothes anxieties, worries...
RES breathing	the ideal winter friction, stops chills, colds, flu, bronchitis, asthma...
RHU pain relief	relieves pains, drains kidneys, anti-rhumatism and joints' pain....
VIT vitality	tonic and vitality the ideal morning friction, increases punch and dynamism for students, sportsmen and exams time.

106 hair	hair regenerative, helps regrowth, tonifies tired limp, brittle, toneless hair.
107 brilliant feast	tissue regenerative, strong "anti-wrinkle" with rose EO. A genuine brilliant feast for all types of skin.
108 feet	circulation, excessive perspiration, heavy legs, hot feet, itching, cellulite, headache, disturbed periods.
CEL cellulite	heavy, swollen, tired legs. difficult circulation, hot and cold feet. In association with 108.
DIG digestion	distending, slow and difficult digestion. "miracle" cure for flatulence.
MIN slimming	elimination, weight control, drains liver, gall bladder.
HAR harmony	the friction harmoniser of physical, mental and spiritual. helps with meditation, balance and creativity.

- 20 drops are sufficient as friction, morning and evening, on solar plexus, nape, spine and sole of feet (except 106, 107 and 108 and CEL).
- One 15 ml bottle = 6 weeks's treatment, morning or evening.

AROMATIC OIL FOR THE FACE

- regenerative and strong "anti-wrinkle".

ABO face, an oil specially designed for the face, is the most wonderful product for face care and all types of skin.

It's the ideal beauty product for all alike, man and women!

*If the skin "absorbs" creams for care
we should ideally be able to "eat" beauty products.
You can with ABO.*

frictions/face oil 101

preparation

- 10 ml wheatgerm oil
- 20 ml St John's wort oil
- 10 ml sesame oil
- 15 ml EO rosewood
- 1 ml EO of rose

apply regularly morning and evening.

NOTE: - *the regenerative "anti-wrinkle" treatment, mroning and evening, 3 weeks*
   - *Men enjoy it too !*
   - *107 friction (see: Frictions) 5 to 7 drops patting*
   - *The aromatic oil ABO (face) is not greasy: light, fine, rich in EO, regenerative in vitamins E, it penetrates immediately.*
   - *for tired blotchy skins:*
     hydrosol of sage + friction 107 + ABO face
   - *for acne skins: hydrosol of cedar + friction 107 + ABO face or ABO tonic.*

NOTE: *peeling may occur during the first 10 days of use: it's not worrying, half dead cells are elimintaed faster and the new skin appears finer, nourished and regenerated.*
   this is the powerful effect of this "super" anti-wrinkle treatment.

Aromatic oil for the outline of the eyes

   - the best product for the eyes is wheatgerm oil.
   - one secret: open a capsule of WGO and apply tapping.
   - it's the cheapest and most efficient method on the market !

ABO eye outline: tonifies
- WGO 90 ml
- SJWO 5 ml
- EO lavender 5ml
- EO rose 1/2 drop
- EO rosewood 8ml

- should red spot appear (as often on fragile eye outline) split this composition with 100 ml WGO.

AROMATIC OIL FOR THE HAIR

- to improve dry hair an oil bath before shampoo.
  leave for 4 to 12 hours.

Preparation

100 ml coco oil, 30 ml WGO, 10 ml EO ylang-ylang
5 ml cedar, 3ml EO thyme, 5ml EO sage.
shake before use, massage scalp well and length of hair. Olive oil
can replace coco or wheatgerm oil.

Note:　　106 friction is applied to the scalp and aromatic oil for
massage treatment is completed with hydrosol of cedar
as a daily lotion.

Note 2:　for hair loss
106 friction +hydrosol of cedar + thyme + sage + live
yeast + draining of liver (horseradish and artichoke
juice) for 3 to 6 weeks

Note 3:　hair rinse after shampoo:
hydrosol of camomile: for blond hair
hydrosol of cedar: disentagle and softens
hydrosol of cedar + sage + thyme + lavender : for all
types of hair.

Note 4:　against lice: rose geranium 10 ml, lavender 10 ml,
sage 10 ml thuya 5 ml.
20 drops in the evening for 7 days
then once a week for 3 weeks.

AROMATIC OIL FOR THE FEET

- to relieve "heated", perspiring red feet.

Preparation:

- 20 ml WGO, 80 ml sesame or olive or almond oil.
  3 ml EO mint, 15 ml EO lavender, 5 ML sage.
- fingi, cold feet, hot feet see Frictions 108 feet.
- hydrosol of mint refreshes.

AROMATIC OIL FOR NAILS

- to re-vitalise brittle, fragile, broken, soft nails.

Preparation:

- Oil bath 5 to 10 min/day for 1 to 3 weeks.
  1 tble sp olive oil + lemon juice + 1 drop EO lemon.
- take trace elements, horsetail of nettle juice, both re-mineralisers

FUMIGATIONS

Before face care and spraying.

They are a preparation for the skin (face, neck and bust) prior to receiving treatment, mask or a regenerative phial.

Preparation:

Fumigation is the association of a few drops of essential oils to hot water steam.

At home use a veryhot water bowl, an inhalator without a nozzle, a "vapomask" or a container of very hot water to which you will add the selected EO.

Put your face above the container and cover your head with towel, just as with a steam bath or an inhalation, this for 3   4 minutes.

Before care, to dilate the pores:

5 to 10 drops of mix.

all skins : EO juniper, cedar or sassafras.

acne skins : EO juniper, cedar or lemon, sassafras or thyme lemon

During or after care : to make the pores close :

dry skins : EO lavender + rosewood + rose-geranium

acne skins : EO lavender + rosewood + lemon

wrinkled skins : EO rosemary + rosewood + sandal

flushed skins : EO cypress + lavender + rosewood

itchy skins : EO rosewood + lavender + camomile

all skins : EO sage.

MASKS

Masks with honey, mud and EO cleanse and smooth the face.

PREPARATION:

1) Honey mask formula:
In 3 table spoons of honey, add 1 to 5 drops of essential oils selected for their desired effect. Mix.
Apply to the face, neck and bust with a wooden spatula.
Keep for about 7 minuts, rinse with warm water.

2) Mudpack formula:
In 3 table spoons of fine clay, green, pink or white, add 1 to 2 drops of essential oils suitable for your skin.
Apply to the face. Keep for 3 to 7 minutes while relaxing.
As soon as the mask dries, re-apply water or remove with warm water.
Follow with an application of tonic, rejuvenative phial or cream, according to your needs, or special aromatic oil for the face.

3) Greasy skin formula:
In 2 spoons of non)heated honey, add 2 drops of essential oil of lemon and 10 drops of essential oil of lavender, apply 7 to 10 minutes.

Cleansing mask
EO sassafras 3 drops, EO lavender 6 drops. Add in 2 tble sp on non- heated honey.

All skins mask
2 drops EO lemon; Mix in powdered clay, green, pink of white with enough water to obtain a slightly thick paste.
Apply to skin 7 to 10 minuted, rinse with water.

Anti-wrinkle mask
EO rosemary, rosewood: 3 drops of each
Add in 2 tble sp of honey, keep for 5 minutes.
Rinse with warm, then cold water.

AFTER SHAVE

Natural, alcohol-free, rejuvenative and "anti-wrinkle".

ABO tonic   60 ml HGB, 30 ml HM, 1 ml EO rose, 20 ml rosemary, 10 ml EO lavender, 1/2 EO vervain, apply a few drops as a non-fat oil nourishes skin

EO lavender   healing, soothes razor rash:
a few drops on skin.

Lavender hydrosol   non greasy, calms, refreshes.

Aquaderma lotion   hydrosols of lavender, sage, thyme, camomile, wild rose
soothes, relaxes.
to be followed with a few drops of ABO tonic or ABO face.

Nota: men enjoy the fresh and tonic fragrance of EO.

Nota 2:   ABO face and aromatic oil are used frequently for face care see ABO.

PERFUMES

Incense fragrance of the senses....
all perfumes are composed of essences
they are the "foundation" of perfumes.

Ingredients: 70% alcohol, a perfume fixative, some EO

Preparation: - 1 to 15 ml of your own EO mixture: your "foundation".
- 100 ml of 70 degrees alcohol
- 1 tinted glass bottle
- mix
- add 2 drops EO sclarified sage: a natural fixative
- leave to rest for 15 days, away from light and heat.
- filter .... then use.

Nota: The same foundation 1 to 15 ml mixed to 250 ml alcohol will produce a toilet water.

Sclarified sage EO is a natural vegetable fixative.

Amber, musk and civet were ans still are used in perfumery as a fixative.

Today fixatives are often synthetically produced.

Advice and Recipes:

-In your "foundation" sparingly use the following EO, as they are strongly olfactive: cinnamon, bergamot, clove, thyme, ginger, origano, mint.....

To compose your "foundation", called "base" in France, country of perfumes
- Select soft and flowery EO: lavender, vervain, rosewood, sandalwood, lemon,rose geranium, ylang-ylang.
- Add drop by drop (and write them down) EO which inspire you. For strong essences simply 1/20th of the original foundation (clove, cinnamon, neroli, rose, ginger ......)
- Dont forget to write down you composition!

Example no 1   : soft, feminine, captivating foundation

Foundation   : rose geranium 7 ml, vervain 4 ml, cedar 3 ml

    add   : 20 drops of essence rose

    add   : 5 drops of essence of sage as fixative.

Rose geranium, vervain and rose have close fragrances which reinforce each other within the same range.

Example no 2   : heady, oriental, suave foundation

Foundation   : sandalwood 10 ml, cedar 5 ml

    add   : 5 drops of essence of sage as fixative

    add   : a few drops of lemon to refresh this oriental foundation or a few drops of ylang-ylang.

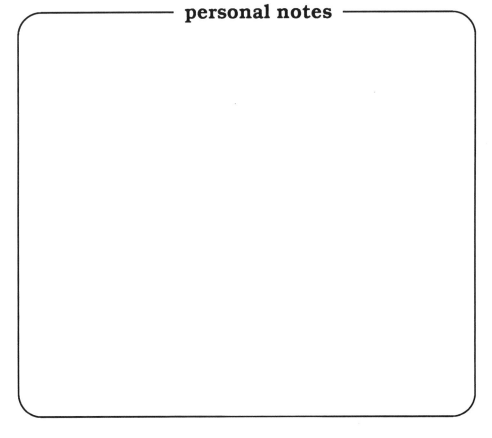

personal notes

FACE TONICS

They are prepared with hydrosols, also called hydrolats or floral waters.

Vie Arôme's hydrosols are produced from the first 20 litres of water from each distillation of aromatic plants, non treated and distilled with spring water.

How to use them?

For the face	rejuvenative, tonic for all skins
	lavender, thyme, rosemary, sage, wild rose, carrot, cedar, camomile and aquaderma....
For razor rash	lavender, rosemary.
For dermatosis and scars	cedar or wild rose + lavender
For hair	softens, silkens: thyme, cedar
	regrowth :cedar
	after sun :thyme, cedar
	blond hair :camomile or camomile + thyme
For baths	(2 tble sp/bath)
soothing child bath	: lavender, camomile
tonic bath	: thyme, rosemary
happy bath	: vervain
For eyes softening	: cornflour water
For eyes relief	: camomile hydrosol

Some advice on usage

lotions	ideal dry skin lotion	: lavender + rosemary + thyme or wild rose + camomile
	ideal wrinkle lotion	: rosemary + sage + lavender or aquaderma or wild rose + lavender.
	ideal acne lotion	: cedar + thyme + lavender or cedar only
	ideal lotion for all skins	: aqauderma

ideal lotion for irritated
skins   : lavender + camomile

And more...

as aftershave   : rosemary hydrosol + lavender
as after sun   : mint hydrosol + lavender +
                                 rosemary

for heavy legs   : mint hydrosol
hair rinse   : cedar hydrosol + thyme
blond hair   : camomile

personal notes

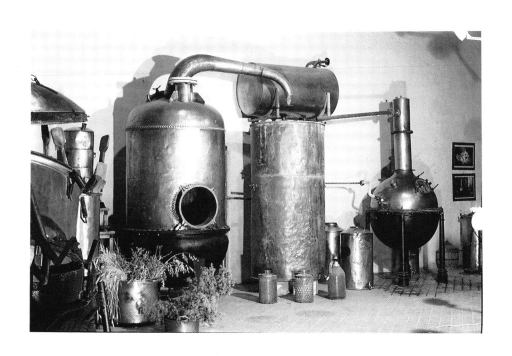

Reconstruction of a distillation factory.
Nineteenth century Musée des Arômes et du parfum
13700 Graveson en Provence

CHAPTER 4

ESSENTIAL OILS IN "COOKING"

- compose your own "culinary pharmacy"

- summary table: EO in the kitchen

- Recipes

    . cocktails with vegetable juice
    . aromatic oils
    . seasonings
    . caviar or vegetable "pâtés"

- hydrosols: natural drinks

- natural "toddies".

COMPOSE YOUR OWN
"CULINARY PHARMACY"

EO*   lemon, orange, mandarin, cinnamon, ginger, bergamot
for "healthy" sweets, pureed fruit.

EO   basil, tarragon, coriander
sauces for salads and germinated seeds

EO   rosemary, marjoram, juniper, nutmeg, sage
for cooked dishes, cereals and vegetable pâtés

EO   savory, cinnamon, thyme, rosemary, coriander, lemon, mint.
for natural toddies, healthy drinks.

Hydrosols mint
for sugarless cordials for children.

Hydrosols vervain, sage, origano, savory, rosemary, juniper
for hot or cold healthy drinks.

EO : Essential Oil

SUMMARY TABLE
ESSENTIAL OILS IN THE KITCHEN

	EO	hydrosol	sweets	in salt dishes	warm drinks	"healty" drinks hydrosols	fresh drinks syrups	aromatic oils for salad
basil	•			•				•
bergamot	•		•		•			
cinnamon	•		•		•			
caraway	•		•	•				
celery	•	•				•		
lemon	•		•		•		• EO	
coriander	•		•	•	•			•
cumin	•			•				
tarragon	•	•		•		•		•
fennel		•				•		
juniper	•	•		•		•		
rose geranium	•		•		•			
ginger	•		•		•			
clove	•				•			
mandarin	•		•		•		• EO	
marjoram	•	•		•	•			•
mint	•	•	•		•	•	• hyd	
nutmeg	•		•					•
origano	•	•		•	•	•	• hyd	
orange	•		•		•		• EO	
parsley		•		•		•		
rosemary	•	•		•	•	•		•
sage	•	•		•	•	•	• hyd	•
savory	•	•		•	•	•	• hyd	•
thyme	•	•		•	•	•		
vervain	•	•	•		•	•	• hyd	

- EO of garlic and onion are never used in cookery :
    the fresh vegetables themselves are full of fragrance
- EO of rose is rarely used: its price matches gold!
- EO of fennel and dill are not used on the market.
- this table takes into account the capacity to "eat or drink" EO or hydrosol.
For example: as hot or cold drink: all EO and hydrosols can be used;
however, as noted, some are more pleasant than others.

RECIPES

COCKTAILS WITH VEGETABLE JUICE

1.EXOTIC COCKTAILS
- **Andalousian:**   tomato, cucumber, pepper + 1 drop EO mint.
- **Carribean:**   carrot, pepper + lime juice (fresh)
- **Mexican:**   carrot, tomato, pepper + lime juice (fresh) + pimento water + 1 drop EO ginger.
- **Indian:**   carrot, green cabbage + 1 drop EO cinnamon.
- **African:**   carrot, cabbage, courgette + 1 drop EO coriander + 1 drop EO caraway
- **Provence:**   carrot, tomato + 1 drop of EO basil.
- **Hawian:**   (very strong) carrot, courgette, pepper + 1 tble sp of decoction (ginger) + 1 sm. sp. pimiento water.

2. COCKTAILS FROM THE FRENCH PROVINCES
- **Midi:**   carrot, celery + 1 drop EO basil or coriander.
- **Basque:**   carrot, tomato, cucumber + 1 drop of EO nutmeg.
- **Alsace:**   carrot, green cabbage + 1 drop EO caraway.
- **Riviera:**   carrot, celery, cucumber + 1 drop EO tarragon.

3. CLEANSING COCKTAILS
- **Excellent for the liver:** carrot 3/4, radish 1/4 + 1 drop EO rosemary
- **Excellent for the kidneys:** carrot 1/2, celery 1/2 + 1 drop EO juniper.
- **Excellent for the tummy:** carrot 1/3, green cabbage 1/3, potato 1/3.

4. TO HELP WITH SUCKLING AND CLEANSING KIDNEYS: fennel.

5. TO REDUCE GENERAL ACIDITY AND LOSE WEIGHT : watermelon or carrot/watermelon.

Summing up: For 1 litre of vegetable juice: 3 to 4 drops of EO.

- The carrot or tomato base in half, the other vegetables for the other half.
  Only radish is to be added with 5 to 10 small radishes or 5cm of horseradish to 1 litre of carrot juice.
  Onion: 1/4 onion per carrot litre.

- Strong vegetables are added in small quantity: celery, radish, leek, onion potato: 1 tble sp per glass of juice.
- to add EO (3/4 drops per litre of juice): place the EO on top of the vegetables in the liquidiser.

- Seasoning (herbal, ginger, saffron or pimento water) is done when serving.
- A vegetable juice can be kept from 4 to 5 hours in a refrigerator. Stir before serving.

- There is no limit in drinking vegetable juices (1 or 2 litres per day without any problem, during a course).
  Remember: they "densify", re-mineralise, tonify and nourish.

- Vegetable juices are real food.
- You can take a few months' course of a simple diet of vegetable juices.

- Treatment with vegetable juices is supreme in cases of serious illness.

- The pause "aperitif of vegetable juice" is sacred just as with traditional drinks it brings: calm, relaxation, smiles.

* Single diet: take one single daily food, several times a day.

* Abbreviation:	tble sp.	table spoon
	sm. sp.	small spoon
	EO	Essential Oil

AROMATIC OILS WITH EO
Prepare 1/4 of first cold pressed olive oil to which are added: 6 drops EO basil or EO coriander or EO tarragon or EO caraway or EO cumin (3 drops only) + fresh pimiento and sea salt (optional) or herbamare.
To be used as a regular oil for salads.
E.O. basil, caraway, cumin, coriander, juniper, rosemary, mountain savory, bay leaf, tarragon, nutmeg, marjoram, origano, can be added 1 drop in the sauce for each handful of germinated seeds per person and for 4 people.

Note: the oil can be replaced in full or in part with yoghurt, cream cheese or avocado.

SEASONINGS
Sea salt with oil, tamarisk, yeast, vegetable extract (powder), pimento, cider vinegar, lemon, lime, paprika, blend well with sauces for germinated seeds.

Other seasonings worth mentioning :
Sunflower seeds soaked (15 mins), hazelnut or almond powder, olive purée... give much variety in seasonings.

"CAVIARS" OR VEGETABLE PATES
A good way not to waste 2/3 days' old seeds:
Put in the mixer germinated seeds with some vegetable juice (carrot, fennel, courgette...), add olive oil and yeast. Season with fresh herbs, basil, tarragon, parsley, garlic, onion... and/or some EO and serve fresh, rapidly.

Recipes and aroma dosage for 6 persons

- whilst cooking :
Cumin, caraway, coriander, nutmeg, thyme, marjoram, sage, rosemary to be added to dosage of 4/8 drops.

Example :
- In couscous : add 1 drop juniper, 2 drops cumin, 1 drop caraway.

- In sauerkraut: add 4 drops juniper, 1 drop caraway, 1 drop coriander.

- In stews (vegetable or meat) : thyme, bayleaf, sage and rosemary will compete in proportions of less than 8 drops.

When serving :
Correct your seasoning with salt, pepper, pimento, curry, saffron, according to the dish and add 1 or 2 drops maximum. They will give the finishing touch to your dish.

This last minute's essential oils will bring out the fullness of their aroma as they are not excessively heated.

HYDROSOLS
SOME ADVICE ON THEIR USE

Quality
Vie Arôme's hydrosols are produced from the first 20 litres of water of each distillation of aromatic plants. These have not been treated and are distilled with spring water. They are natural floral waters.

HOW TO USE THEM?

On the face :
- Rejuvenator, tonic for all skins : lavender, thyme, rosemary, sage, carrot,cedar, camomile and aquaderma.....

Razor rash:
lavender, rosemary.
Dermatosis and scars : cedar.

Hair:
- soften: thyme, cedar.
- growth: cedar
- after sun: thyme: cedar
- blond hair:camomile.

Bath:
(2 tble sp/bath)
soothing child bath: lavender, camomile.
Tonic bath:
thyme, rosemary, origano, savory.
It's an hydrosol not EO which is liable to "burn".

Eyes:
- soothing:cornflour water.
- relief: camomile

Drink:
they are the new "liquid" herbal teas and the "specific hygienic day drink".
sage, mint, origano, thyme, eucalyptus, juniper .....

2 tble sp in 1 li. 1/2 water/day or 1 sm. sp/cup of non-boiling or not ice cold water.

Cooking
add to vegetable juices, soups, seasonings, salad dressings, sorbets ...

"Hydrosol" is a specific name given by nelly grosjean for specific "natural floral water" or "hydrolat".

aromatherapie Vie' Arôme
la chevêche - petite route du grès
13690 - graveson en provence
france
tel: 90 95 81 72 - fax:90 95 85 20

NATURAL "TODDIES" WITH E.O.

A: **Anti-flu and tonic:**
Origano, thyme, cinnamon, clove, rose geranium, ginger (optional), 1 drop of each on a large spoon of honey, juice of lemon and a large cup of hot water. Can be taken 2/3 times a day without any problem.

Anti-cough:
Pine, eucalyptus, orange, 1 drop of each on a spoonful of honey, very hot water and lemon juice.
If necessary, drink 2/3 times per day.

Memory cocktail:
Clove, coriander, rosemary, 1 drop of each, in a large glass of water and 1 mint honey spoonful.

Asthma cocktail:
Thyme, hyssop, camomile, cajeput, A drop of each on a spoonful of honey, warm water, serve with ice cubes.

Anti-tobacco cocktail:
Sassafras, sage, rose geranium, marjoram, lavender, 1 drop of each in a spoonful of honey and a large glass of warm water served with ice cubes and a dash of mint cordial.

Aphrodisiac cocktail:
Savory, Ceylon cinnamon, clove, rosemary, rose geranium, 1 drop of each on a spoonful of honey in a glass of warm water, to be served with ice cubes as a long drink, a dash of mint syrup can complete this cocktail.

B. **Anti-indigestion Drinks:**
Clove, ginger, origano, 1 drop of each on a spoonful of honey and in a large glass of warm water, every 2 hours.

C. **Refreshing drinks:**
Cedar, rose geranium or lemon: 1 drop of each on a spoonful of honey in a large glass of warm or cold water.

personal notes

Life is joy."
Giono

"Joy is proof that what you live is good.""
Hindu saying

"Joy is all, it's up to us to discover it.""
Confucius.

A place to visit and gather information on aromatherapy, perfumes and natural medicines, between the Alpilles and the Montagnette, close to les Baux de Provence, in the heart of the countryside.

1) biological cultivation of aromatic plants..

2) distillation of essential oils and hydrosols.

3) Vie' Arôme's aromatherapeutic laboratory: production and distribution, mail order, (france and abroad).

4) health school and lectures open to the public

5) advice, consultation, lectures and training in aromatherapy and holistic medicine, naturopathy, rolfing and geobiology (team of therapists).

6) musée des arômes et du parfum: free conducted tours for groups or individuals.

7) aromatherapy and perfume shop: for sales to visitors.

8) publishing of note books and books: mental and physical medicine.

9) health food restaurant in the main house "mas", lunch, tea, or healthy natural drinks.

nelly grosjean - la chevêche - tél. 90 95 81 55 / 90 95 85 20

GREEN SEED EXPLORATION
Save our planet 92

An expedition in search of disappearing plants in the tropical forests.

WHY?
To save and protect the health capital of our planet.

This expedition is associated to the 1992 Save the Planet Movement whose first world congress will be held in Rio de Janeiro next June.

It will bring together associations, movements and foundations concerned with the protection of our planet, of our environment, our earth, plants, animals from pollution.
Amongst the organisations taking part: Foundation Cousteau, Greenpeace, Save the Alps, The Aga Khan Foundation, Greenwave, World Wildlife Fund (WWF), UNESCO, World Health Organisation (WHO), PNU environment, World Watch Institute.

They will all meet with one goal: to save our planet and leave our children and future generations, a clean, living earth.

GREEN SEED EXPLORATION was initiated by Wayne Christenson, an American ethnologist, scientist and philosopher.

In order to finance other similar expeditions with identical goals, the association du musée des arômes et du parfum (graveson, france), in the heart of Provence, together with nelly grosjean, is participating in the sponsorship of this expedition.

GOALS
To collate, classify and create a data bank library of genetic codes for seeds and plants under all forms, and analyse their specific properties.

126

These plants have been used by the Australian Aborigines, and this for the past 40,000 years, to heal, cure, energise physical or mental abilities.

The first Green Seed Exploration will take place in Australia, this will be followed by a second expedition in New Guinea, then Central Africa and lastly, the Amazon : four barely known tropical forests.

Started in January 1992, this programme will spread every four to six years.

The gathering of collected data could lead to pharmaceutical laboratories and oher similar concerns, to enlarge their natural pharmacopia.

Today, the public and the medias are much open to the use of natural medicines and the return to "natural" things in all areas is increasing too.

Green Seed Exploration's european contact is at the musée des arômes et du parfum in graveson in provence.

For all additional information, offers of help, support participation, please contact:

musée des arômes et du parfum
département green seed exploration
13690 graveson en provence - france
tel: 90 95 81 55 - fax 90 95 85 20

All proceeds from the sale of this book will be donated to "green seed exploration".

Visit the musée des arômes et du parfum
graveson en provence

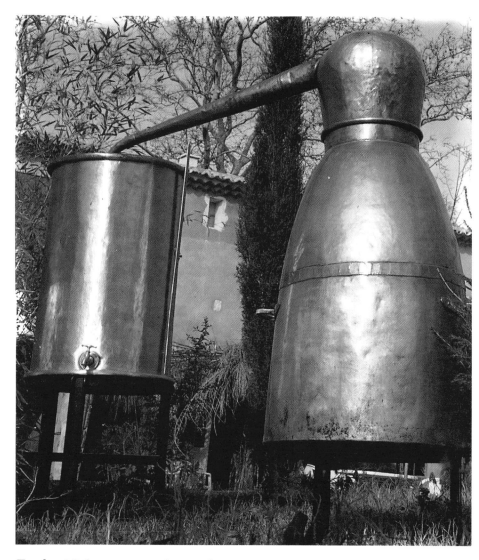

Early 19th century lavender cupper steel known as "Tête de
Maure" (Moor's head), Muséee des arômes et du parfum,
13690 - graveson en provence - france.

La chevêche
petite route du grès   13690 graveson
tel 90 95 81 55 - fax 90 95 85 20

Achevé d'imprimer sur les presses
de l'imprimerie GROUPE 3
16, rue du Génie 13003 Marseille

I.S.B.N. 2 - 950 4286 - 3 - 0